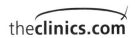

SLEEP MEDICINE CLINICS

Medical Disorders and Sleep

Guest Editor
NANCY A. COLLOP, MD

March 2007 • Volume 2 • Number 1

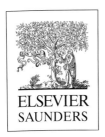

An imprint of Elsevier, Inc
PHILADELPHIA LONDON TORONTO MONTREAL SYDNEY TOKYO

W.B. SAUNDERS COMPANY
A Division of Elsevier Inc.

1600 John F. Kennedy Boulevard • Suite 1800 • Philadelphia, PA 19103-2899

http://www.sleep.theclinics.com

SLEEP MEDICINE CLINICS Volume 2, Number 1
March 2007 ISSN 1556-407X, ISBN-13: 978-1-4160-4367-6 ISBN-10: 1-4160-4367-5

Editor: Sarah E. Barth

The ideas and opinions expressed in *Sleep Medicine Clinics* do not necessarily reflect those of the Publisher. The Publisher does not assume any responsibility for any injury and/or damage to persons or property arising out of or related to any use of the material contained in this periodical. The reader is advised to check the appropriate medical literature and the product information currently provided by the manufacturer of each drug to be administered to verify the dosage, the method and duration of administration, or contraindications. It is the responsibility of the treating physician or other health care professional, relying on independent experience and knowledge of the patient, to determine drug dosages and the best treatment for the patient. Mention of any product in this issue should not be construed as endorsement by the contributors, editors, or the Publisher of the product or manufacturers' claims.

Sleep Medicine Clinics (ISSN 1556-407X) is published quarterly by W.B. Saunders Company, 360 Park Avenue South, New York, NY 10010-1710. Months of publication are March, June, September and December. Business and editorial offices: 1600 John F. Kennedy Boulevard, Suite 1800, Philadelphia, PA 19103-2899. Accounting and circulation offices: 6277 Sea Harbor Drive, Orlando, FL 32887-4800. Periodicals postage paid at New York, and additional mailing offices. Subscription prices are $129.00 per year (US individuals), $50.00 (US students), $259.00 (US institutions), $149.00 (Canadian individuals), $85.00 (Canadian and foreign students), $279.00 (Canadian institutions), $149.00 (foreign individuals), and $279.00 (foreign institutions). Foreign air speed delivery is included in all *Clinics* subscription prices. All prices are subject to change without notice. POSTMASTER: Send address changes to *Sleep Medicine Clinics,* Elsevier Periodicals Customer Service, 6277 Sea Harbor Drive, FL 32887-4800. **Customer Service: 1-800-654-2452 (US). From outside of the United States, call 1-407-345-4000. E-mail: hhspcs@wbsaunders.com**.

Reprints: For copies of 100 or more, of articles in this publication, please contact the Commercial Reprints Department, Elsevier Inc., 360 Park Avenue South, New York, New York 10010-1710. Tel.: (212) 633-3813, Fax: (212) 462-1935, e-mail: reprints@elsevier.com.

Printed in the United States of America.

GOAL STATEMENT

The goal of *Sleep Clinics of North America* is to keep practicing physicians up to date with current clinical practice by providing timely articles reviewing the state of the art in patient care.

ACCREDITATION

The *Sleep Clinics of North America* is planned and implemented in accordance with the Essential Areas and Policies of the Accreditation Council for Continuing Medical Education (ACCME) through the joint sponsorship of the University of Virginia School of Medicine and Elsevier. The University of Virginia School of Medicine is accredited by the ACCME to provide continuing medical education for physicians.

The University of Virginia School of Medicine designates this educational activity for a maximum of 15 *AMA PRA Category 1 Credits*™. Physicians should only claim credit commensurate with the extent of their participation in the activity.

The American Medical Association has determined that physicians not licensed in the US who participate in this CME activity are eligible for 15 *AMA PRA Category 1 Credits*™.

Credit can be earned by reading the text material, taking the CME examination online at http://www.theclinics.com/home/cme, and completing the evaluation. After taking the test, you will be required to review any and all incorrect answers. Following completion of the test and evaluation, your credit will be awarded and you may print your certificate.

FACULTY DISCLOSURE/CONFLICT OF INTEREST

The University of Virginia School of Medicine, as an ACCME accredited provider, endorses and strives to comply with the Accreditation Council for Continuing Medical Education (ACCME) Standards of Commercial Support, Commonwealth of Virginia statutes, University of Virginia policies and procedures, and associated federal and private regulations and guidelines on the need for disclosure and monitoring of proprietary and financial interests that may affect the scientific integrity and balance of content delivered in continuing medical education activities under our auspices.

The University of Virginia School of Medicine requires that all CME activities accredited through this institution be developed independently and be scientifically rigorous, balanced and objective in the presentation/discussion of its content, theories and practices.

All authors/editors participating in an accredited CME activity are expected to disclose to the readers relevant financial relationships with commercial entities occurring within the past 12 months (such as grants or research support, employee, consultant, stock holder, member of speakers bureau, etc.). The University of Virginia School of Medicine will employ appropriate mechanisms to resolve potential conflicts of interest to maintain the standards of fair and balanced education to the reader. Questions about specific strategies can be directed to the Office of Continuing Medical Education, University of Virginia School of Medicine, Charlottesville, Virginia.

The authors/editors listed below have identified no professional or financial affiliations for themselves or their spouse/partner:

Strahil T. Atanasov, MD, DAPN, DABSN; Sarah Barth (Acquisitions Editor); Peter T.P. Bye, MBBS, PhD; William J. Calhoun, MD, FCCP; Timothy A. Connolly, MD; Patrick Hanly, MD, FRCPC, DABSM; Susan M. Harding, MD; Vidya Krishnan, MD; Teofilo Lee-Chiong, MD (Consulting Editor); Margaret D. Lineberger, PhD; Louise McGrath, RMN; Melanie K. Means, PhD; Vahid Mohensin, MD; Babak Mokhlesi, MD, MSc; Amanda J. Piper, PhD; Steven Reid, MB, PhD, MRCPsych; and, Amir Sharafkhaneh, MD.

The authors/editors listed below identified the following professional or financial affiliations for themselves or their spouse/partner:

Helen J. Burgess, PhD is a consultant for Respironics and Physicians Information and Education Resource.

Sean M. Caples, DO receives a research grant from ResMed Foundation and Restore Medical.

Nancy A. Collop, MD (Guest Editor) is an independent contractor for Sepracor; and is on the advisory board/committee for the Sleep Services of America and Johns Hopkins Pharmaquip.

Jack D. Edinger, PhD is an independent contractor for Helicor, Inc. and Respironics; is a consultant for Sepracor; and is on the speaker's bureau for the Sleep Medicine Education Institute.

Ronald R. Grunstein, MD, PhD has undertaken sponsored research for: Cypress Bioscience, Cephalon, Sanofi-Aventis, and GSK.

Mary Ip, MD is an invited speaker at a Consensus Conference organized by International Diabetes Federation (IDF); ResMed Ltd provides an unrestricted educational grant for this conference.

Virend K. Somers, MD, DPhil is a consultant for Cardiac Concepts, and is an independent contractor for ResMed Foundation.

Edward J. Stepanski, PhD is an independent contractor for Takeda Pharmaceuticals and is on the speaker's bureau for Sanofi-Aventis.

Disclosure of Discussion of non-FDA approved uses for pharmaceutical products and/or medical devices:

The University of Virginia School of Medicine, as an ACCME provider, requires that all faculty presenters identify and disclose any "off label" uses for pharmaceutical and medical device products. The University of Virginia School of Medicine recommends that each physician fully review all the available data on new products or procedures prior to instituting them with patients.

TO ENROLL

To enroll in the Sleep Clinics of North America Continuing Medical Education program, call customer service at 1-800-654-2452 or visit us online at www.theclinics.com/home/cme. The CME program is available to subscribers for an additional fee of $99.95.

MEDICAL DISORDERS AND SLEEP

CONSULTING EDITOR

TEOFILO LEE-CHIONG JR., MD
Head, Section of Sleep Medicine, National Jewish
Medical and Research Center, Denver; Associate
Professor of Medicine, University of Colorado
Health Sciences Center, Denver, Colorado

GUEST EDITOR

NANCY A. COLLOP, MD
Associate Professor of Medicine, Johns Hopkins
University, Division of Pulmonary and Critical
Care Medicine, Baltimore, Maryland

CONTRIBUTORS

STRAHIL T. ATANASOV, MD
Assistant Professor of Medicine, Division of
Allergy, Pulmonary, Immunology, Critical Care,
and Sleep [APICS]

HELEN J. BURGESS, PhD
Assistant Professor of Behavioral Sciences,
Rush University Medical Center, Chicago,
Illinois

PETER T.P. BYE, MBBS, PhD
Associate Professor, Department of Respiratory
and Sleep Medicine; Director, Cystic Fibrosis Unit,
Royal Prince Alfred Hospital, Camperdown and
Cystic Fibrosis Group, Woolcock Institute of
Medical Research, University of Sydney, Sydney,
Australia

WILLIAM J. CALHOUN, MD
Sealy and Smith Distinguished Professor,
Vice Chairman for Research, Department
of Internal Medicine, University of
Texas Medical Branch, Galveston,
Texas

SEAN M. CAPLES, DO
Assistant Professor of Medicine, Mayo Clinic
College of Medicine; Consultant, Division of
Pulmonary and Critical Care Medicine,
Department of Medicine, Mayo Clinic, Rochester,
Minnesota

NANCY A. COLLOP, MD
Associate Professor of Medicine,
Johns Hopkins University, Division of
Pulmonary and Critical Care Medicine,
Baltimore, Maryland

TIMOTHY A. CONNOLLY, MD
Baylor College of Medicine Pulmonary/Critical
Care Section, Houston, Texas

JACK D. EDINGER, PhD
Clinical Professor, Department of Psychiatry
and Behavioral Sciences, Duke University
Medical Center; Senior Psychologist,
Veterans Affairs Medical Center (116B),
Durham, North Carolina

RONALD R. GRUNSTEIN, MD, PhD
Professor, Department of Respiratory
and Sleep Medicine, Royal Prince
Alfred Hospital, Camperdown;
Director, Sleep and Circadian Group,
Woolcock Institute of Medical Research,
University of Sydney,
Sydney, Australia

PATRICK HANLY, MD, FRCPC, D ABSM
Professor of Medicine, University of
Calgary; Director, Sleep Centre,
Foothills Medical Centre, Calgary,
Alberta, Canada

SUSAN M. HARDING, MD
Professor of Medicine and Medical Director,
UAB Sleep-Wake Disorders Center, Division of
Pulmonary, Allergy, and Critical Care Medicine,
University of Alabama at Birmingham,
Birmingham, Alabama

MARY IP, MD
Professor of Medicine, Division of Respiratory
and Critical Care Medicine, Department of
Medicine, The University of Hong Kong,
Queen Mary Hospital, Pokfulam,
Hong Kong, China

VIDYA KRISHNAN, MD
Pulmonary/Critical Care Fellow, Johns Hopkins
University, Division of Pulmonary and
Critical Care Medicine, Baltimore, Maryland

MARGARET D. LINEBERGER, PhD
Research Associate, Department of Psychiatry and
Behavioral Sciences, Duke University Medical
Center, Durham, North Carolina

LOUISE McGRATH, RMN
Clinical Nurse Specialist in Psychiatry, Department
of Liaison Psychiatry; and Department of HIV
Medicine, St Mary's Hospital, London, United
Kingdom

MELANIE K. MEANS, PhD
Research Associate, Department of Psychiatry
and Behavioral Sciences, Duke University
Medical Center; Clinical Psychologist, Veterans
Affairs Medical Center (116B), Durham,
North Carolina

VAHID MOHSENIN, MD
Professor of Medicine, Section of Pulmonary and
Critical Care Medicine, and Director, Yale Center
for Sleep Medicine, Yale University School of
Medicine, New Haven, Connecticut

BABAK MOKHLESI, MD, MSc
Assistant Professor of Medicine,
Section of Pulmonary and Critical Care; Director,
Sleep Disorders Center, The University
of Chicago Pritzker School of Medicine,
Chicago, Illinois

AMANDA J. PIPER, PhD
Senior Physiotherapist, Respiratory Failure
Service, Department of Respiratory
and Sleep Medicine, Royal Prince
Alfred Hospital, Camperdown; and
Research Fellow, Woolcock Institute of Medical
Research, University of Sydney, Australia

STEVEN REID, MB, PhD
Consultant Psychiatrist, Department
of Liaison Psychiatry, St Mary's Hospital,
London, United Kingdom and;
Honorary Senior Lecturer,
Department of Psychological Medicine,
Imperial College, London,
United Kingdom

AMIR SHARAFKHANEH, MD
Veterans Affairs Medical Center, Houston, Texas;
Baylor College of Medicine, Houston, Texas

VIREND K. SOMERS, MD, DPhil
Professor of Medicine, Mayo Clinic
College of Medicine; Consultant,
Division of Cardiovascular Diseases and
Division of Hypertension,
Department of Medicine,
Mayo Clinic, Rochester, Minnesota

EDWARD J. STEPANSKI, PhD
Accelerated Community Oncology Research
Network, Memphis, Tennessee

MEDICAL DISORDERS AND SLEEP

Volume 2 • Number 1 • March 2007

Contents

> COPD is the fourth leading cause of death in the US, affecting 14 millions adults. Symptoms related to sleep disturbances are common in individuals with moderate to severe COPD, particularly in elderly patients. One cause of morbidity in this population is abnormalities in gas exchange and resultant hypoxemia, which can lead to elevated pulmonary pressures, dyspnea, and right ventricular overload and failure. Sleep has profound adverse effects on respiration and gas exchange in patients with COPD. Smoking cessation, bronchodilation, inhaled steroids in those with a reversible component, and pulmonary rehabilitation are cornerstones of treatment. Improvement in lung mechanics and gas exchange should lead to better sleep quality and health status.

> Sleep-related asthma, also known as *nocturnal asthma*, is characterized by a decrease in forced expiratory volume in 1 second of at least 15% between bedtime and wake-up time in patients diagnosed with asthma. In some patients, these decrements in lung function can reach 50%. Nocturnal asthma seems to have significant clinical impact, and the most recent United States guidelines for asthma management emphasize that nocturnal symptoms indicate the need for more aggressive controller therapy. Several factors have been proposed to cause or worsen nocturnal bronchoconstriction, including horizontal posture in bed, airway cooling, exposure to allergens, gastro-esophageal reflux, obesity, and obstructive sleep apnea. Several mechanisms of nocturnal bronchial spasm have also been proposed, including circadian fluctuations in hormone levels, circadian variations in autonomic nervous system activity, airway inflammation, and genetic predisposition.

Sleep and Glucose Intolerance/Diabetes Mellitus   19

Mary Ip and Babak Mokhlesi

> The sleep state itself has modulatory effects on glucose homeostasis. Epidemiologic and experimental studies suggest that sleep loss and sleep disturbances are detrimental to metabolic function and may predispose to obesity or glucose intolerance. Apart from the common risk factor of obesity, increasing data also support that obstructive sleep apnea exerts independent adverse effects on glucose intolerance and diabetes mellitus, although definitive evidence is still needed.

Sleep Disturbance in Fibromyalgia   31

Margaret D. Lineberger, Melanie K. Means, and Jack D. Edinger

> Fibromyalgia (FM), characterized by diffuse myalgia, multiple topographically specific tender points, chronic fatigue, psychosocial distress, and disturbed, unrefreshing sleep, is a significant health problem. Clinical survey studies suggest that the majority of FM patients present with insomnia complaints, including difficulty initiating sleep, sleep maintenance problems, or persistent nonrestorative sleep. Studies of clinical FM patients have shown that a worsening of sleep enhances subsequent daytime distress and pain complaints, whereas exacerbations of daytime pain or psychosocial distress often are followed by increased nocturnal sleep disruption. Given such findings, it seems reasonable to speculate that sleep disturbance is mechanistically important to the etiology or symptom maintenance of the FM syndrome. This article provides an overview of FM-related sleep difficulties and their treatment.

Gastroesophageal Reflux During Sleep   41

Susan M. Harding

> Esophageal acid clearance is markedly delayed during sleep and requires an arousal response for clearance. The prevalence of sleep-related gastroesophageal reflux (GER) is 79% in GER patients and approximately 25% in the Sleep Heart Health Study participants. Sleep-related GER is associated with esophagitis, Barrett's esophagus, esophageal adenocarcinoma, arousals, poor sleep quality, excessive daytime sleepiness, impaired quality of life, and extraesophageal manifestations of GER. The possible association between GER and obstructive sleep apnea is currently being investigated. Diagnosis of sleep-related GER includes careful history taking and esophageal pH testing, which can also be integrated with polysomnography. Treatment includes conservative measures, medications (primarily proton pump inhibitors, H_2 receptor antagonists, and prokinetic agents), and surgical fundoplication in selected patients.

HIV/AIDS   51

Steven Reid and Louise McGrath

> Insomnia is common in people living with HIV and AIDS. Evidence to date suggests that there is no consistent relationship between altered sleep architecture and disease progression. The exception is late-stage HIV infection associated with cognitive impairment. The antiretroviral drug efavirenz has also been found to be a contributor but the most significant risk factor is psychological morbidity. This highlights the importance of investigation and management of underlying anxiety and depression in people presenting with persistent insomnia.

Sleep Disorders and End-Stage Renal Disease 59

Patrick Hanly

Sleep complaints and sleep disorders are common in patients with end-stage renal disease (ESRD). Patients frequently report both insomnia and excessive sleepiness, which are significant contributors to their impaired quality of life. Restless legs syndrome, periodic limb movement disorder, and sleep apnea are highly prevalent. In addition to causing sleep disruption and sleep loss, these conditions may further increase the considerable cardiovascular morbidity and mortality in this patient population. Although conventional dialysis does not correct these sleep disorders, nocturnal hemodialysis and renal transplantation may be more effective.

Sleep and Cancer 67

Edward J. Stepanski and Helen J. Burgess

Patients with cancer commonly report disturbed sleep, fatigue, and daytime drowsiness. Although sleep disturbance contributes to significantly reduced quality of life, the overall significance of poor sleep at it relates to fatigue, pain, depression, or other health outcomes is unknown. Given that management of these symptoms is desirable for optimal outcomes in the treatment of cancer, evaluation and treatment of sleep disturbance in patients undergoing treatment for cancer is important. Given the need to minimize treatment burden, evaluation and treatment of sleep disturbance in this population may require clinical protocols specifically designed for patients with cancer. Further investigation is also needed into the role of pro-inflammatory cytokines as either a cause or consequence of sleep disturbance in this population.

Sleep, Blood Pressure Regulation, and Hypertension 77

Sean M. Caples and Virend K. Somers

The link between sleep and the cardiovascular system is well recognized, both in health and disease. Because of the relative ease of noninvasive ambulatory measurement, no aspect of this relationship has been more studied than blood pressure (BP). The study of obstructive sleep apnea has furthered the understanding of blood pressure and its regulatory mechanisms. More recently, as the scientific and public eyes have focused on inadequate sleep as a plague of modern society, research efforts have been directed at the consequences of sleep debt on systemic disease, including blood pressure dysregulation.

Sleep and Breathing in Cystic Fibrosis 87

Amanda J. Piper, Peter T.P. Bye, and Ronald R. Grunstein

Sleep hypoxemia, hypoventilation, and cough occur in patients with CF, especially as pulmonary disease worsens. Sleep disturbance is common, with a significant number of patients reporting their sleep quality to be poor. Changes in neurocognitive function and daytime activation may be related to sleep loss. Improvements in gas exchange have been achieved during acute physiological and short-term interventional studies with oxygen breathing, while nocturnal noninvasive ventilation has been shown to maintain ventilation in REM sleep and reduce work of breathing. However, high-quality long-term trials examining the impact of these therapies on disease progression and daytime function are lacking.

Vidya Krishnan and Nancy A. Collop

> Sleep-related breathing disorders and pulmonary hypertension (PH) are inextricably linked, although the mechanisms of association are complex. Physiologic changes associated with sleep-related breathing disorders, including hypoxia, hypercoagulability, and systemic inflammation, may result in alterations in pulmonary hemodynamics. While sleep-disordered breathing in and of itself may not result in severe PH, it likely results in elevated pulmonary arterial pressures. Treatment of sleep-disordered breathing appears to improve pulmonary arterial pressures. Data are needed to determine if the treatment of sleep-disordered breathing will improve clinical outcomes of patients with PH.

Timothy A. Connolly and Amir Sharafkhaneh

> This article reviews cardiovascular physiology and ventilatory control during sleep, the epidemiology of sleep-related breathing disorder (SRBD) in congestive heart failure (CHF), the pathophysiology of central sleep apnea (CSA) as it relates to CHF, and the clinical features and implications of SRBD in systolic CHF. It then focuses on treatment options for CHF-related CSA including continuous positive airway pressure and newer modalities such as adaptive pressure support servo-ventilation.

SLEEP
MEDICINE
CLINICS

Sleep Med Clin 2 (2007) xi–xii

Foreword

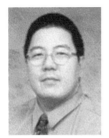

Teofilo Lee-Chiong Jr., MD
Consulting Editor

Teofilo Lee-Chiong Jr., MD
Section of Sleep Medicine
National Jewish Medical and Research Center
Denver, CO 80206, USA

E-mail address:
lee-chiongt@njc.org

Much of our knowledge of normal human physiology, medical disorders, and the effect of pharmacologic therapy on these diseases is based largely on research conducted while subjects were awake. The influence of sleep on medical disorders is just beginning to be appreciated by clinicians and researchers. Sleep, or its lack, and the influences of circadian rhythm can alter the presentation and adversely affect the symptoms of a variety of medical conditions, including respiratory, cardiac, gastrointestinal, renal, rheumatologic, and infectious disorders. Conversely, many medical disorders can disturb sleep and alter sleep architecture.

Chronic obstructive pulmonary disease can give rise to complaints of insomnia or excessive sleepiness. It can lead to frequent nighttime awakenings and nonrestorative sleep secondary to nocturnal coughing or dyspnea. Nocturnal hypoxemia and hypercapnia can develop, especially in patients who have severe disease or comorbid obstructive sleep apnea syndrome (OSA), so-called "overlap syndrome." Oxygen desaturation occurs during periods of hypoventilation, which is worse during rapid eye movement sleep. Sleep in patients who have nocturnal asthma is characterized by poor sleep quality with frequent arousals caused by coughing, dyspnea, wheezing, and chest discomfort. Complaints of insomnia and/or excessive daytime sleepiness are common. As in chronic obstructive pulmonary disease, sleep-related hypoxemia can occur during exacerbations of the disease. Frequency of periodic breathing or central apneas during sleep can increase in patients who have diabetes mellitus. There also is an association between glucose intolerance and OSA.

In fibromyalgia, sleep often is described as unrefreshing or nonrestorative, with patients complaining of insomnia and early morning awakenings. In many patients who have fibromyalgia, there is a correlation between poor sleep quality and perception of pain intensity (ie, poor sleepers may report more pain, and those who have greater pain during the daytime may have poorer nighttime sleep). Patients who have gastroesophageal reflux (GER) often report having heartburn symptoms at night that negatively affect sleep quality. Sleep-related GER is associated with more prolonged esophageal acid clearance times. Nocturnal GER

doi:10.1016/j.jsmc.2007.01.003

seems to be common in patients who have OSA, and continuous positive airway pressure therapy decreases the frequency of nocturnal GER symptoms in these patients.

HIV infection and sleep are closely interrelated, with many patients complaining of insomnia, recurrent arousals, and excessive sleepiness. Sleep disturbance can be aggravated further by antiviral therapy. Common sleep complaints of patients receiving maintenance hemodialysis for end-stage renal disease include insomnia, prolonged awakenings, and excessive sleepiness. Patients who have end-stage renal disease also may have a higher likelihood of developing OSA, restless leg syndrome, periodic limb movement disorder, and reversal of day-night sleep patterns.

Cystic fibrosis often is accompanied by poor sleep quality, sleep fragmentation, and nighttime episodes of coughing. Oxygen desaturation can occur. These sleep-related parameters are correlated with physiologic variables of disease severity and can worsen during disease exacerbations. Finally, sleep and sleep disorders influence the course of hypertension and cancer, and are, in turn, affected by them.

The bidirectional nature of the relationship between sleep and medical disorders is evident throughout the various articles of this issue of *Sleep Medicine Clinics*. Thus, an understanding of the daytime consequences of medical disorders must be accompanied by an appreciation of the role of sleep on disease course and prognosis.

SLEEP
MEDICINE
CLINICS

Sleep Med Clin 2 (2007) xiii

Preface

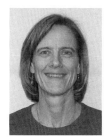

Nancy A. Collop, MD
Guest Editor

Nancy A. Collop, MD
Johns Hopkins University
Division of Pulmonary and Critical Care Medicine
1830 East Monument St., Room 555
Baltimore, MD 21205, USA

E-mail address:
ncollop@jhmi.edu

Sleep medicine has come a long way since MacNish in 1934 stated: "sleep is the intermediate state between wakefulness and death; wakefulness … the active state of all the animal and intellectual functions, and death as that of their total suspension." Over the past 50 years we have learned that sleep is not close to death at all but is a different state of being. Moreover, the states within sleep, rapid eye movement and non–rapid eye movement, are as different from each other as sleeping is from waking. As we have begun to learn more about sleep, further revelations regarding its substantial impact on diverse medical conditions have become apparent. This issue of *Sleep Medicine Clinics* explores the impact of sleep and sleep disorders on a variety of common medical disorders.

The choice of medical disorders included in this issue was based on the amount of medical literature available. For thousands of medical disorders the data on sleep effects are scant. The disorders included here have more substantial data, although most authors point out the need for more research.

The topics chosen are diverse and represent diseases found in millions of patients throughout the world. The authors likewise are from a variety of locations throughout the world and represent a particular area of expertise in both the medical condition described and in the field of sleep medicine. The diverse topics range from respiration and esophageal function during normal sleep to chronomodulated chemotherapy and alpha EEG sleep anomaly. The topics highlight the substantial impact that sleep and its disorders can have on the individual patient and stress the need for practitioners caring for such patients to be cognizant of these issues. This issue should be excellent reading for sleep practitioners and also for primary care and specialist practitioners caring for the diverse patient populations described. I am grateful to the authors who devoted their time and talent to writing the various articles.

I dedicate this book to my parents, Barb and Bill Abbey, whose love and encouragement have inspired me throughout my career.

1556-407X/07/$ – see front matter © 2007 Elsevier Inc. All rights reserved.
sleep.theclinics.com

doi:10.1016/j.jsmc.2007.01.002

SLEEP
MEDICINE
CLINICS

Sleep Med Clin 2 (2007) 1–8

Sleep in Chronic Obstructive Pulmonary Disease

Vahid Mohsenin, MD

Chronic obstructive pulmonary disease (COPD) is the fourth leading cause of death with increasing frequency in the general population. It is estimated that approximately 14 million people in the United States have COPD. The prevalence of COPD in men aged 20 to 69 years is about 14% [1,2]. The increased prevalence and mortality from COPD is occurring worldwide and is attributed to rise in cigarette smoking and environmental pollution. In addition to these potent extrinsic factors, there appears to be a strong genetic predisposition for the development of clinically significant airflow obstruction such that it occurs in only approximately 15% of smokers.

COPD is characterized by chronic airway obstruction that is not fully reversible. Pathologically, the term COPD encompasses the following entities: (1) chronic bronchitis with obstruction and inflammation of small airways with mucus and Goblet cell hyperplasia and excess mucus production often referred to as "Blue Bloaters" and (2) emphysema with enlargement of air spaces secondary to destruction of lung parenchyma and consequent loss of elasticity with closure of small airways, commonly known as "Pink Puffers." Although patients with COPD present clinically with either chronic bronchitis or emphysema, most patients have both pathologic conditions to a varying extent and their clinical phenotype is often expressed as what is the dominant underlying pathology.

Patients with COPD mainly die from cardiovascular and respiratory diseases as well as cancer. One major cause of morbidity in this population is abnormalities in gas exchange and resultant hypoxemia. Sleep has profound adverse effects on respiration and gas exchange in patients with COPD.

Respiration during normal sleep

Human sleep can be divided into two patterns, non–rapid eye movement (NREM) sleep and rapid eye movement sleep (REM), each with distinctive

Section of Pulmonary and Critical Care Medicine, Yale Center for Sleep Medicine, Yale University School of Medicine, 40 Temple Street, Suite 3C, New Haven, CT 06510, USA
E-mail address: vahid.mohsenin@yale.edu

doi:10.1016/j.jsmc.2006.11.013

physiologic characteristics. While the time spent in stage 3 and 4 NREM sleep decreases as an individual ages, the percentage spent in REM sleep remains unchanged. These sleep phases have different and distinct effects on respiration in normal humans.

NREM Sleep

There is a reduction in alveolar ventilation from wakefulness to NREM sleep in normal individuals. Accompanying this reduction is a mild increase in arterial CO_2 tensions of 2 to 8 mm Hg with a reciprocal decrease in arterial oxygen tension (PaO_2) with no significant changes in the arterial oxygen saturation (SaO_2). The hypercapnia occurs despite a 10% to 30% fall in metabolic CO_2 production. The fall in ventilation is a result of a small reduction in tidal volume with little or no change in breathing frequency. Apneas are rare in NREM sleep in normal subjects. During NREM sleep there is an approximately 50% decrease in the slope of the CO_2 response line compared with the awake response, as well as rightward shift. The data on the arousal responses to CO_2 are mixed; some have shown no consistent sleep state–related differences in arousal to hypercapnia, while others have shown an increase in arousal responses. The ventilatory response to hypoxia decreases by approximately 33% during NREM sleep. Hypoxia, when induced with a normal arterial CO_2, is a poor stimulus to arousal in normal subjects.

REM sleep

REM sleep comprises 20% to 25% of total sleep time in adults. There is irregularity in respiration with significant breath-to-breath variability and increased mean respiratory frequency compared with NREM sleep. Marked reductions in ventilation with bursts of eye movements in REM sleep in humans have been observed despite increased respiratory frequency in these periods. This supports the observation that the fall of SaO_2 in patients with COPD is more severe in REM sleep periods associated with eye movements (phasic REM) than during periods without eye movements (tonic REM). Carbon dioxide tension during REM sleep increases by 1 to 2 mm Hg compared with NREM sleep; however, it is quite variable. During REM sleep, the CO_2 response decreases further compared with NREM sleep. The mechanism of reduced ventilatory responses in sleep is still unresolved; however, it is likely that the overall fall in response is the combination of reduced reflex drive and an increase of upper airway flow resistive load [3,4]. The ventilatory response to hypoxia decreases by approximately 67% during REM sleep.

Mechanisms of hypoxia during sleep in COPD

Several studies have shown that recurrent transient hypoxemia during sleep is frequent in patients with COPD [5,6]. The nocturnal hypoxemia is particularly marked in "blue and bloated" and frequently occurs during REM sleep. The measurement of minute ventilation with a pneumotachograph and oxygen saturation with a pulse oximeter in a group of patients with severe COPD demonstrated a nearly 20% lower SaO_2 during non-REM sleep and 40% lower oxygenation during REM sleep than during the awake state, primarily because of reduced tidal volume [7]. There are several mechanisms underlying nonapneic oxygen desaturation during sleep. They include decreased functional residual capacity, diminished ventilatory responses to hypoxia and hypercapnia [8,9], impaired respiratory mechanical effectiveness, diminished arousal responses [10], respiratory muscle fatigue [11], diminished nonchemical respiratory drive [8], increase in upper airway resistance [12], and the position of baseline saturation values on the oxyhemoglobin dissociation curve (Box 1) [13].

Decrease in functional residual capacity

Recumbency and sleep are associated with approximately 10% decrease in functional residual capacity (FRC) in healthy subjects [14]. Hudgel and colleagues [15], using respiratory impedance plethysmography to monitor the changes in FRC during sleep in COPD patients, observed more marked oxygen desaturation in those with the greatest reduction in FRC. The reduction in FRC reduces the oxygen gas stores with impairment of gas exchange. These patients also demonstrated a fall in diaphragmatic inspiratory EMG activity. But not all studies have shown reductions in FRC and suggested decreased tidal volume as the primary cause for

---

Box 1: Mechanism of hypoxemia during sleep in COPD

- Decreased functional residual capacity and decreased oxygen stores in the lung
- Hypoventilation

  REM sleep–associated inhibition of respiratory muscles
  Decreased chemosensitivity to arterial carbon dioxide tension ($PaCO_2$) and arterial oxygen tension (PaO_2)
  Increased arousal threshold

- Changes in ventilation-perfusion relationship
- Position of baseline saturation on the oxygen-hemoglobin dissociation curve

hypoxemia and gas exchange abnormality during sleep in COPD [12]. Many subjects remain asleep with arterial saturation as low as 70% with no apparent NREM-REM differences.

Hypoventilation

As stated earlier in this article, ventilation is lower during all stages of sleep because of disappearance of the influence of wakefulness and the change in the respiratory center sensitivity. A detailed assessment of respiratory mechanics during NREM sleep in hypercapnic COPD patients demonstrated increased upper airway resistance with no changes in pulmonary resistance or intrinsic positive end-expiratory pressure ($PEEP_i$), end-expiratory lung volume, or dynamic compliance [16]. However, investigations in nonhypercapnic COPD patients have not shown a more profound decrease in minute ventilation during NREM sleep in COPD patients than in healthy subjects [12,17].

The reduction in ventilation is particularly more pronounced during REM sleep resulting in more severe oxygen desaturation in COPD. The COPD patients are particularly more prone to REM sleep–associated hypoxemia because of the loss of contribution of intercostal respiratory muscles and diminution in diaphragmatic contribution to ventilation in a hyperinflated lung with increased dead space. Furthermore, because many patients with COPD are hypoxemic, with waking arterial oxygen tension at or near the steep portion of the oxyhemoglobin dissociation curve, a given decrease of alveolar ventilation will result in a greater decrease in SaO_2 than in healthy persons.

Changes in perfusion-ventilation relationship

The hypoxemia during REM sleep is associated with little rise in arterial $PaCO_2$ suggesting perfusion-ventilation mismatching [18]. Direct measurements of arterial PaO_2 and $PaCO_2$ during sleep in six COPD patients showed that mean PaO_2 decreased from 51 mm Hg in NREM sleep to 44 mm Hg during REM sleep, whereas $PaCO_2$ increased from 50 mm Hg to 53 mm Hg. Catterall and colleagues [19] also found that the fall in PaO_2 in REM sleep was much greater than the corresponding rise in $PaCO_2$. Although many studies have demonstrated a correlation between awake SaO_2 and oxygen desaturation during sleep in patients with COPD [5,9,20,21], the degree of hypoxemia cannot be predicted from awake measurement of SaO_2 in individual patients with any degree of accuracy because of considerable variance around the regression line [22]. Likewise, pulmonary function testing correlates poorly with nocturnal hypoxemia. The degree of airflow obstruction, as defined by forced

expiratory volume at one second/forced vital capacity (FEV_1/FVC), increases the risk of oxygen desaturation during sleep only when it is less than 65%. In this study, oxygen desaturation was defined as greater than 5% of total sleep time with SaO_2 of less than 90% [23].

Effects of nocturnal hypoxemia on central hemodynamics

Pulmonary arterial pressure increases during sleep in patients with COPD [24,25]. This is related to alveolar hypoxia causing vasoconstriction and increased pulmonary vascular resistance. Pulmonary hypertension and cor pulmonale are commonly seen in patients with COPD and chronic hypoxemia ($PaO_2 < 55$ mm Hg) [26]; however, the clinical importance of hypoxemia during sleep in patients with COPD is unknown. In animal studies modeled after REM-related hypoxemia in COPD, rats that were exposed to 12% oxygen for 2 hours a day for 4 weeks developed significant right ventricular hypertrophy [27]. However, other studies have demonstrated that oxygen does not increase survival in patients with less severe hypoxia [28]. Similarly, in patients with COPD who have nocturnal hypoxemia, nocturnal treatment with oxygen does not appear to increase survival or delay the need for continuous oxygen therapy [29].

Sleep in COPD

Emphysema patients often report difficulty initiating and maintaining sleep, resulting in increased daytime sleepiness. Objectively, patients have increased latencies, shortened total sleep time, and an increased number of nocturnal arousals with increase in light sleep [30,31]. In elderly patients with COPD, both depression and arthritis were the most significant independent correlates for the majority of sleep scores [32]. In severe cases, the sleep disturbance is usually related to nocturnal cough, wheezing, and shortness of breath due to worsening of pulmonary mechanics and gas exchange during sleep. In a large survey of patients with COPD, Klink and colleagues [33] found that with one respiratory symptom (cough or wheezing) present, 39% reported insomnia and 12% excessive daytime sleepiness. With both symptoms present the prevalence of insomnia and excessive daytime sleepiness was 53% and 23%, respectively. Sleep studies in COPD have shown poor-quality sleep as judged by marked increase in sleep stage changes, frequent arousals and awakening, and by decreased total sleep time (summed Stages 2, 3, 4, and REM) with increased number of arousals [30,34]. However, in an adult community setting and part of the Sleep Heart Health Study, Sanders and colleagues [23] found that patients with mild obstructive airway disease (FEV$_1$/FVC 63.8% ± 6.6%, mean ± SD) did not perceived themselves to have excessive daytime sleepiness and had only minimally altered sleep quality and sleep architecture. Lung volume reduction surgery in patients with severe emphysema (FEV1 = 28%) and hyperinflation improved total sleep time and sleep efficiency as well as oxygen saturation during sleep compared with medically treated group [35].

Sleep-disordered breathing in COPD

Because of high prevalence of sleep apnea and COPD in the middle-age population [36], patients with COPD may have concomitant sleep apnea that can further exacerbate their gas exchange during sleep. The term "overlap syndrome" was introduced by Flenley [37] to describe this association. Chaouat and colleagues [38] studied 265 patients who were referred to a sleep laboratory for various reasons and found 11% with obstructive airway disease. These patients were older than the remainder of the group and were all male. The "overlap syndrome" group had lower awake PaO$_2$ and higher PaCO$_2$ and higher pulmonary artery pressure with more marked hypoxemia during sleep than the other group but with no difference in the apnea-hypopnea index. The more significant oxygen desaturation during sleep was, in large part, attributable to lower baseline saturation at the onset of apnea in the overlap group. The main determinants of pulmonary hypertension in the overlap group were daytime arterial blood gases that contributed 30% and FEV$_1$, which contributed 12%. The blunting of ventilatory responsiveness to CO$_2$ in "overlap syndrome" patients may also contribute to abnormality of gas exchange during apneic events [39]. A prospective study by the same French team demonstrated lower 5-year survival in these patients compared with the sleep apnea only group despite similar treatment with continuous positive airway pressure [40].

Indications for sleep studies in COPD

Although there are no specific studies on the prevalence of sleep apnea in COPD, the current data suggest no excess incidence [20,23]. Thus, the indication for polysomnography in patients with COPD is similar to those with sleep-related breathing disorders. However, the presence of polycythemia, cor pulmonale, and neuropsychologic impairment in patients with COPD whose daytime PaO$_2$ is greater than 60 mm Hg would be an indication for sleep study for assessment of nocturnal oxygen desaturation and sleep apnea.

Treatment

Oxygen

Continuous oxygen therapy is the only modality in the management of patients with COPD and hypoxemia (PaO$_2$ ≤ 55 mm Hg) that has been shown to increase survival. In the Nocturnal Oxygen Therapy Trial (NOTT), patients who received continuous oxygen had a 50% decrease in mortality compared with those on a 12-hour regimen [41]. In a controlled prospective study of COPD patients with PaO$_2$ of 55 to 65 mm Hg with severe airflow obstruction (mean FEV$_1$ 0.83 L) no survival benefit was demonstrated with long-term oxygen therapy [28].

Patients with COPD who show substantial desaturation during sleep comprise another group in which long-term oxygen therapy might provide clinical benefits [42]. Increased mortality among patients with nocturnal desaturation and daytime PaO$_2$ = 60 mm Hg has been demonstrated in retrospective studies [43]. However, well-controlled studies have not shown that use of nocturnal supplemental oxygen alters mortality or clinical course in patients who experience hypoxemia only during sleep, other than slightly lowering pulmonary artery pressure [29]. However, other benefits might accrue from improved quantity and quality of sleep. Nocturnal oxygen supplementation has been shown to improve sleep quality in patients with COPD as judged by shorter latency to sleep, increase in REM sleep, as well as stages 3 and 4, and decreased number of arousals [30].

A joint effort by the American Thoracic Society and the European Respiratory Society has updated the 1995 guidelines for the diagnosis and management of COPD, which is currently posted on the Web site of the American Thoracic Society. Following are some of the guidelines and recommendations regarding oxygen therapy:

- Pulse oximetry is a good method for following trends in oxygen saturation and can be used for titrating the oxygen flow setting in stable patients with good circulation.
- Nocturnal oxygen therapy is not recommended for isolated nocturnal hypoxemia except in special circumstances, such as the presence of complications of hypoxemia, ie, polycythemia or cor pulmonale that are not explained by the awake PaO$_2$. Measurement of nocturnal oxygen saturation is recommended in these settings even when the PaO$_2$ is greater than 55 mm Hg. Nocturnal oxygen

should be prescribed to patients who suffer substantial desaturation ($\leq 88\%$) during sleep.

Many patients on chronic supplemental oxygen spend more than 30% of the night with SaO_2 less than 90% while breathing oxygen at the daytime flow rate [42,44]. If the patient does not have sleep-disordered breathing as a result of other causes, the administration of oxygen at a flow rate higher than the daytime setting will usually correct nocturnal hypoxemia. In some patients, particularly those with hypercapnia, higher oxygen flows may induce further carbon dioxide retention with resultant morning headache and confusion. This hazard is best avoided by careful adjustment of the flow of oxygen to maintain the PaO_2 between 60 and 65 mm Hg. In most cases there is no need for nocturnal oximetry or sleep study for titration of oxygen flow rate, except that in the "overlap" group, the administration of continuous positive airway pressure may obviate the need for nocturnal oxygen supplementation.

Inhaled anticholinergic therapy

In a randomized double-blind study of moderate to severe COPD, four weeks of treatment with ipratropium bromide resulted in significant improvement in mean nocturnal SaO_2 and perceived sleep quality with increase in REM sleep time. No significant improvement was noted in other sleep stages or total sleep time [45]. Similarly, in a recent randomized placebo-controlled, double-blind study of 95 patients with severe COPD, the tiotropium group had a higher SaO_2 during REM and during total sleep time compared with placebo without affecting the sleep quality [46].

Theophylline

Oral theophylline has been shown to improve nocturnal oxygen saturation and morning peak flow rates in patients with COPD [47,48]. However, the effect of theophylline on sleep parameters and quality has been variable, some showing improvement [47] and others no significant effect [48,49].

Effect of respiratory muscle training

Sleep is associated with decreased activity of respiratory muscles particularly inspiratory intercostal muscles. Nonobstructive hypoventilation occurs more severely during sleep in patients with COPD because of (1) loss of contribution of intercostal muscles and (2) inability of a mechanically disadvantaged diaphragm to compensate for the latter. In a controlled study, inspiratory muscle training for a period of 10 weeks improved the inspiratory muscle strength and nocturnal oxygen saturation

in a group of 10 patients with stable COPD compared with sham-treated control [50].

Noninvasive ventilation

The utility of noninvasive positive pressure ventilation (NPPV) during acute exacerbation of COPD has been documented [51]. However, there are few studies to examine the effectiveness of NPPV in stable patients with COPD. Uncontrolled studies on a small number of patients have shown that NPPV used at home may improve oxygenation and reduce hospital admissions in patients with severe COPD and hypercapnia [52]. In a controlled crossover study, NPPV in inspiratory support mode was demonstrated to improve sleep efficiency and total sleep time in severe but stable COPD patients with hypercapnia without improvement in gas exchange [53]. A meta-analysis of nocturnal NPPV in patients with stable COPD demonstrated that ventilatory support for 3 months did not improve lung function, gas exchange, or sleep efficiency [53]; however, there may be a subgroup of patients with severe stable COPD who might benefit from NPPV. In response to increasing use of NPPV in COPD patients and conflicting data, the Centers for Medicare and Medicaid Services (CMS) has adopted a series of guidelines based on the recommendation of the National Association for Medical Directors of Respiratory Care and the American College of Chest Physicians consensus conference (   ) [54].

The evidence for beneficial effects of NPPV in "overlap syndrome" is more convincing. In a nonrandomized study on patients with COPD and sleep apnea, treatment of sleep apnea resulted in improvement of arterial blood gases and pulmonary arterial pressure compared with just oxygen supplementation without specific treatment for sleep apnea [38,55]. It, therefore, appears important to diagnose coexisting sleep apnea and treat it appropriately. The combination of NPPV and long-term oxygen therapy may be more effective, but larger control studies are needed. In our Center, patients with "overlap syndrome" receive NPPV first to improve their sleep apnea–hypopnea syndrome unless there is hypoxemia during wakefulness. In this situation they will be treated with low-flow oxygen to maintain SaO_2 between 87% and 90% before they receive NPPV for sleep apnea.

Hypnotics and COPD

Hypnotics, particularly benzodiazepines, could adversely affect respiration and gas exchange in patients with COPD. These agents decrease the upper airway muscle tone increasing the airway resistance and may blunt the respiratory drive.

Box 2: Guidelines for use of noninvasive positive pressure ventilation in severe stable COPD

Consensus conference guidelines*
Symptomatic after optimal therapy
Sleep apnea excluded
$PaCO_2 \geq 55$ mm Hg or
$PaCO_2$ 50–54 mm Hg and evidence of nocturnal hypoventilation based on nocturnal oximetry showing sustained desaturation to <89% for $\geq$ 5 minutes while patient is on his or her usual FiO_2
Repeated hospitalization

Centers for Medicare and Medicaid Services guidelines
$PaCO_2 \geq 52$ mm Hg and
Evidence of nocturnal hypoventilation based on nocturnal oximetry showing sustained desaturation to <89% for $\geq$ 5 minutes while patient is on his or her usual FiO_2
Sleep apnea excluded clinically (polysomnogram not required)
Requisite 3-month initial trial of bi-level device without a back-up rate

FiO_2, fraction of inspired oxygen

* Adapted from Clinical indications for noninvasive positive pressure ventilation in chronic respiratory failure due to restrictive lung disease, COPD, and nocturnal hypoventilation—a consensus conference report. Chest 1999;116:521–534.

However, there is evidence that some hypnotics, such as zolpidem, can be used in less severe COPD without significant adverse effects on gas exchange [56].

References

[1] Petty TL, Pierson DJ, Dick NP, et al. Follow-up evaluation of prevalence for chronic obstructive bronchitis and chronic airway obstruction. Am Rev Respir Dis 1976;114:881–90.

[2] Lebowitz MD. The trends in airway obstructive disease morbidity in the Tucson epidemiologic study. Am Rev Respir Dis 1989;140:S35–41.

[3] Henke KG, Dempsey JA, Kowitz JM, et al. Effects of sleep-induced increases in upper airway resistance on ventilation. J Appl Physiol 1990;69(2):617–24.

[4] Morrell MJ, Harty HR, Adams L, et al. Changes in total pulmonary resistance and PCO_2 between wakefulness and sleep in normal human subjects. J Appl Physiol 1995;78(4):1339–49.

[5] Catterall JR, Douglas NJ, Calverley PM, et al. Transient hypoxemia during sleep in chronic obstructive pulmonary disease is not a sleep apnea syndrome. Am Rev Respir Dis 1983;128(1):24–9.

[6] Douglas NJ. Nocturnal hypoxemia in patients with chronic obstructive pulmonary disease. Clin Chest Med 1992;13(3):523–32.

[7] Becker HF, Piper AJ, Flynn WE, et al. Breathing during sleep in patients with nocturnal desaturation. Am J Respir Crit Care Med 1999;159:112–8.

[8] Kelsen SG, Fleegler B, Altose MD. The respiratory neuromuscular response to hypoxia, hypercapnia and obstruction to airflow in asthma. Am Rev Respir Dis 1979;120:517–27.

[9] Littner MR, McGinty DJ, Arand DL. Determinants of oxygen desaturation in the course of ventilation during sleep in chronic obstructive pulmonary disease. Am Rev Respir Dis 1980;122(6):849–57.

[10] Phillipson EA. Control of breathing during sleep. Am Rev Respir Dis 1978;118:909–39.

[11] Grassino A, Macklem PT. Respiratory muscle fatigue and ventilatory failure. Annu Rev Med 1984;35:625–47.

[12] Ballard RD, Clover CW, Suh BY. Influence of sleep on respiratory function in emphysema. Am J Respir Crit Care Med 1995;151:945–51.

[13] Wynne JW, Block AJ, Hemenway J, et al. Disordered breathing and oxygen desaturation during sleep in patients with chronic obstructive pulmonary disease. Chest 1978;73(Suppl 2):301–3.

[14] Hudgel DW, Devodatta P. Decrease in functional residual capacity during sleep in normal humans. J Appl Physiol 1984;57:1319–22.

[15] Hudgel DW, Martin RJ, Capehart M, et al. Contribution of hypoventilation to sleep oxygen desaturation in chronic obstructive pulmonary disease. J Appl Physiol 1983;55:669–77.

[16] O'Donoghue FJ, Catcheside PG, Eckert DJ, et al. Changes in respiration in NREM sleep in hypercapnic chronic obstructive pulmonary disease. J Physiol 2004;559(Pt 2):663–73.

[17] Meurice JC, Marc I, Series F. Influence of sleep on ventilatory and upper airway response to CO_2 in normal subjects and patients with COPD. Am J Respir Crit Care Med 1995;152(5 Pt 1):1620–6.

[18] Fletcher EC, Levin DC. Cardiopulmonary hemodynamics during sleep in subjects with chronic obstructive pulmonary disease. The effect of short and long-term oxygen. Chest 1984;85:6–14.

[19] Catterall JR, Calverley PMA, MacNee W, et al. Mechanism of transient nocturnal hypoxemia in hypoxic chronic bronchitis and emphysema. J Appl Physiol 1985;59:1698–703.

[20] Connaughton JJ, Catterall JR, Elton RA, et al. Do sleep studies contribute to the management of patients with severe chronic obstructive pulmonary disease? Am Rev Respir Dis 1988;138:341–4.

[21] Little SA, Elkholy MM, Chalmers GW, et al. Predictors of nocturnal oxygen desaturation in patients with COPD. Respir Med 1999;93(3):202–7.

[22] Mohsenin V, Guffanti EE, Hilbert J, et al. Daytime oxygen saturation does not predict

nocturnal oxygen desaturation in patients with chronic obstructive pulmonary disease. Arch Phys Med Rehabil 1994;75:285–9.

[23] Sanders MH, Newman AB, Haggerty CL, et al. Sleep and sleep-disordered breathing in adults with predominantly mild obstructive airway disease. Am J Respir Crit Care Med 2003;167:7–14.

[24] Coccagna G, Lugaresi E. Arterial blood gases and pulmonary and systemic arterial pressure during sleep in chronic obstructive pulmonary disease. Sleep 1978;1:117–24.

[25] Boysen PG, Block AJ, Wynne JW, et al. Nocturnal pulmonary hypertension in patients with chronic obstructive pulmonary disease. Chest 1979;76:536–42.

[26] Tarpy SP, Celli BR. Long-term oxygen therapy. N Engl J Med 1995;333:710–4.

[27] Moore-Gillon JC, Cameron IR. Right ventricular hypertrophy and polycythemia in rats after intermittent exposure to hypoxia. Clin Sci (Lond) 1985;69:595–9.

[28] Gorecka D, Gorzelak K, Sliwinski P, et al. Effect of long-term oxygen therapy on survival in patients with chronic obstructive pulmonary disease with moderate hypoxemia. Thorax 1997; 52:674–9.

[29] Chaouat A, Weitzenblum E, Kessler R, et al. A randomized trial of nocturnal oxygen therapy in chronic obstructive pulmonary disease patients. Eur Respir J 1999;14:1002–8.

[30] Calverley PMA, Brezinova V, Douglas NJ, et al. The effect of oxygenation on sleep quality in chronic bronchitis and emphysema. Am J Respir Crit Care Med 1982;126: 206–10.

[31] Cormick W, Olson LG, Hensley MJ, et al. Nocturnal hypoxaemia and quality of sleep in patients with chronic obstructive lung disease. Thorax 1986;41(11):846–54.

[32] Bellia V, Catalano F, Scichilone N, et al. Sleep disorders in the elderly with and without chronic airflow obstruction: the SARA study. Sleep 2003;26: 318–823.

[33] Klink ME, Dodge R, Quan SF. The relation of sleep complaints to respiratory symptoms in a general population. Chest 1994;105:151–4.

[34] Fleetham J, West P, Mezon B, et al. Sleep, arousal, and oxygen desaturation in chronic obstructive pulmonary disease. The effect of oxygen therapy. Am Rev Respir Dis 1982;126(3):429–33.

[35] Krachman SL, Chatila W, Martin UJ, et al. Effects of lung volume reduction surgery on sleep quality and nocturnal gas exchange in patients with severe emphysema. Chest 2005;128(5):3221–8.

[36] Young T, Palta M, Dempsey J, et al. The occurrence of sleep disordered breathing among middle-aged adults. N Engl J Med 1993;328:1230–5.

[37] Flenley DC. Sleep in chronic obstructive lung disease. Clin Chest Med 1985;6:651–61.

[38] Chaouat A, Weitzenblum E, Krieger J, et al. Association of chronic obstructive pulmonary disease and sleep apnea syndrome. Am J Respir Crit Care Med 1995;151(1):82–6.

[39] Radwan L, Maszczyk Z, Koziorowski A, et al. Control of breathing in obstructive sleep apnoea and in patients with the overlap syndrome. Eur Respir J 1995;8:542–5.

[40] Chaouat A, Weitzenblum E, Krieger J, et al. Prognostic value of lung function and pulmonary haemodynamics in OSA patients treated with CPAP. Eur Respir J 1999;13:1091–6.

[41] Nocturnal Oxygen Therapy Trial Group. Continuous or nocturnal oxygen therapy in hypoxemic chronic obstructive lung disease: a clinical trial. Ann Intern Med 1980;93:391–8.

[42] Fletcher EC, Luckett RA, Goodnight-White S, et al. A double-blind trial of nocturnal supplemental oxygen for sleep desaturation in patients with chronic obstructive pulmonary disease and a daytime PaO_2 above 60 mmHg. Am Rev Respir Dis 1992;145:1070–6.

[43] Kimura H, Suda A, Sakuma T, et al. Nocturnal oxyhemoglobin desaturation and prognosis in chronic obstructive pulmonary disease and late sequelae of pulmonary tuberculosis. Intern Med 1998;37:354–9.

[44] Plywaczewski R, Sliwinski P, Nowinski A, et al. Incidence of nocturnal desaturation while breathing oxygen in COPD patients undergoing long-term oxygen therapy. Chest 2000;117: 679–83.

[45] Martin RJ, Bucher B, Becki L, et al. Effect of ipatropium bromide treatment on oxygen saturation and sleep quality in COPD. Chest 1999; 115:1338–45.

[46] McNicholas WT, Calverley PM, Lee A, et al. Long-acting inhaled anticholinergic therapy improves sleeping oxygen saturation in COPD. Eur Respir J 2004;23:825–31.

[47] Mulloy E, McNicholas WT. Theophylline improves gas exchange during rest, exercise and sleep in severe chronic obstructive pulmonary disease. Am Rev Respir Dis 1993;148:1030–6.

[48] Mann GC, Chapman KR, Ali SH, et al. Sleep quality and nocturnal respiratory function with once-daily theophylline (Uniphyl) and inhaled salbutamol in patients with COPD. Chest 1996; 110:648–53.

[49] Martin RJ, Pak J. Overnight theophylline concentrations and effects on sleep and lung function in chronic obstructive pulmonary disease. Am Rev Respir Dis 1992;145:540–4.

[50] Heijdra YF, Dekhuijzen PN, van Herwaarden CL, et al. Nocturnal saturation improves by target-flow inspiratory muscle training in patients with COPD. Am J Respir Crit Care Med 1996; 153:260–5.

[51] Antonelli M, Conti G, Rocco M, et al. A comparison of noninvasive positive pressure ventilation and conventional mechanical ventilation in patients with acute respiratory failure. N Engl J Med 1998;339:429–35.

[52] Jones SE, Packham S, Hebden M, et al. Domiciliary nocturnal intermittent positive pressure ventilation in patients with respiratory failure due to severe COPD: long-term follow-up and effect on survival. Thorax 1998;53:495–8.

[53] Krachman SL, Quaranta AJ, Berger TJ, et al. Effects of noninvasive positive pressure ventilation on gas exchange and sleep in COPD patients. Chest 1997;112:623–8.

[54] Clinical indications for noninvasive positive pressure ventilation in chronic respiratory failure due to restrictive lung disease, COPD, and nocturnal hypoventilation—a consensus conference report. Chest 1999;116:521–34.

[55] Fletcher EC, Schaaf M, Miller J, et al. Long-term cardiopulmonary sequelae in patients with sleep apnea and chronic lung disease. Am Rev Respir Dis 1987;135:525–33.

[56] Steens R, Pouliot Z, Millar T, et al. Effects of Zolpidem and Triazolam on sleep and respiration in mild to moderate chronic obstructive pulmonary disease. Sleep 1993;16:318–26.

SLEEP
MEDICINE
CLINICS

Sleep Med Clin 2 (2007) 9–18

The Relationship Between Sleep and Asthma

Strahil T. Atanasov, MD[a], William J. Calhoun, MD[b],*

Asthma

Approximately 300 million people worldwide currently have asthma, and its prevalence increases by 50% every decade. In North America, 10% of the population has asthma. Worldwide, approximately 180,000 deaths annually are attributable to asthma, although overall mortality rates have decreased since the 1980s. In different Western countries, the financial burden on patients who have asthma ranges from $300 to $1300 per patient per year [1]. Sleep-related asthma, also known as *nocturnal asthma*, is characterized by a decrease in forced expiratory volume in 1 second (FEV_1) of at least 15% between bedtime and wake-up time in patients diagnosed with asthma. In some patients, these decrements in lung function can reach 50% [2].

Epidemiology of sleep-related asthma

The 1988 study on the prevalence of nocturnal asthma symptoms by Turner-Warwick [3] included 7729 outpatients who had asthma. It showed that approximately 40% of patients experienced asthma symptoms every night, 64% reported awakening with symptoms at least three times a week, and 74% awoke with asthma symptoms at least once a week. In a study of 3129 patients who had nocturnal asthma, Dethlefsen and Repgas [4] concluded that approximately 94% of dyspneic episodes occurred between 10:00 PM and 7:00 AM, and that 4:00 AM was when the highest frequency of symptoms occurred. A newer study in 2006 included 13,493 patients who had persistent asthma. The prevalence of nocturnal symptoms was still high

[a] Division of Allergy, Pulmonary, Immunology, Critical Care, and Sleep (APICS), Route 0561, 301 University Blvd., Galveston, TX 77555, USA
[b] Department of Internal Medicine, 301 University Boulevard, University of Texas Medical Branch, Galveston, TX 77555, USA
* Corresponding author.
E-mail address: william.calhoun@utmb.edu (W.J. Calhoun).

1556-407X/07/$ – see front matter © 2007 Elsevier Inc. All rights reserved.
sleep.theclinics.com

doi:10.1016/j.jsmc.2006.12.001

at 60% [5]. Therefore, the high prevalence of nocturnal symptoms is well established in patients who have asthma.

Consequences of sleep-related asthma

Nocturnal asthma is believed to indicate uncontrolled asthma, but it also has important effects on quality-of-life (QOL) and psychometric indexes [6]. In a study of more than 400 children who had asthma and their parents, Diette and colleagues [7] at Johns Hopkins University showed that 40% of children had experienced nighttime awakening within the previous 4 weeks. Moreover, children who experienced nocturnal awakenings also had an increased number of days of school missed, increased symptom severity, and an increased use of reliever medications. In addition, the parents of these children who had nocturnal asthma had an increased frequency of missed work days. Thus, nocturnal asthma impacts the QOL of both patients and their families.

An earlier study by Weersink and colleagues [8] showed similar findings. More than 40 asthmatic subjects underwent psychometric testing before and after randomized treatment with inhaled fluticasone, inhaled salmeterol, or a combination of these agents. At baseline, subjects who had asthma showed various psychometric abnormalities compared with controls. However, each treatment strategy was associated with an improvement in psychometric indices (to the normal range of findings) and pulmonary function. No differences among the strategies were observed for the outcomes measured.

A study by Stores and colleagues [9] showed that children who had asthma experienced significantly more disturbed sleep, tended to have more psychological problems, and performed less well on some tests of memory and concentration than matched controls. In general, improvement of nocturnal asthma symptoms caused by changes in treatment was followed by improvement in sleep and psychological function in subsequent weeks. These data provide another important rationale for identifying and treating nocturnal asthma. Thus, nocturnal asthma seems to have significant clinical impact, and the most recent United States guidelines for asthma management [10] particularly emphasize that the presence of nocturnal symptoms indicate the need for more aggressive controller therapy.

Circadian alterations in lung function and airway responsiveness

Healthy humans and those who have asthma have two peaks of maximal sleepiness during the 24-hour period: 4:00 AM and 4:00 PM, which vary in circadian fashion. Lung function has also been shown to fluctuate over the 24-hour period in both healthy individuals and those who have asthma, with peak lung function occurring at 4:00 PM and minimal lung function at 4:00 AM. Both the peak and trough of lung function coincide with the sleepiest times of the 24-hour period. These fluctuations are distinctively more pronounced in patients who have nocturnal asthma; they exhibit decrements in FEV_1 between 4:00 PM and 4:00 AM of more than 15% (Fig. 1) [11].

Sleep is the major synchronizer of circadian fluctuations in lung function. A study by Hetzel and Clark [12] on the effects of sleep interruption and deprivation showed that the circadian rhythm of peak expiratory flow rate (PEFR) is often in phase with the timing of sleep. The same authors concluded that circadian variation of asthma in shift workers was intimately related to sleep and independent of solar time [13]. If sleep in general is the main synchronizer of lung function diurnal variations, the next question would be whether any particular stage of sleep is more frequently associated with nocturnal asthma attacks. A study by Kales and colleagues [14] did not support the hypothesis that asthmatic episodes were specifically related to rapid eye movement (REM) sleep; these episodes were randomly distributed throughout the stages of sleep in proportion to the amount of time spent in each sleep stage.

Not only is lung function at its minimum at 4:00 AM but also the airway is both hyperreactive and underresponsive to bronchodilators in individuals who have nocturnal asthma. Individuals who have nocturnal asthma display increased airway hyperresponsiveness at 4:00 AM if compared

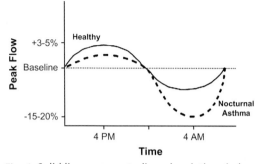

Fig. 1. Solid line represents diurnal variations in lung function of healthy individuals. Dotted line represents diurnal variations in lung function in nocturnal asthma sufferers. The difference between the two is most pronounced at their nadir at around 4:00 AM. (*From* Sutherland ER. Nocturnal asthma. J Allergy Clin Immunol 2005;116(6):1179–86; with permission from American Academy of Allergy, Asthma, and Immunology.)

with an awake daytime baseline. This finding was shown in a study by decreasing the methacholine PC_{20} FEV_1 (concentration required to induce a 20% decrease in FEV_1) from 1.80 ± 0.75 mg/mL at 4:00 PM to 0.47 ± 0.16 mg/mL at 4:00 AM [15].

Inhaled bronchodilators improve bronchoconstriction in many patients who have nocturnal asthma, but this response is somewhat blunted at 4:00 AM. A study evaluating the albuterol dose–response at night in patients who had nocturnal asthma showed a slower response to albuterol and a higher dose required because more severe airway obstruction was present on awakening [16].

Factors causing or worsening bronchoconstriction during sleep

Several factors have been proposed to cause or worsen nocturnal bronchoconstriction, including horizontal posture in bed, airway cooling, exposure to allergens, gastroesophageal reflux, obesity, and obstructive sleep apnea (OSA).

Regarding horizontal posture, a study by Whyte and Douglas [17] strongly suggested that the supine posture is not an important cause of overnight bronchoconstriction. Clark and Hetzel [13] showed that patients who have asthma who lie in bed throughout the 24-hour period preserve their circadian pattern of rising PEFR during the day.

Cold air is a well-known trigger of bronchial spasm in individuals who have asthma. Breathing cooler air at night may play a role in causing nocturnal bronchospasm. At least one study on the effect of breathing warm, moisturized air (36°C–37°C, 100% saturation) compared with room air (23°C, 17%–24% saturation), suggested that airway cooling, which occurs also as a consequence of body cooling, plays a significant role in triggering nocturnal asthma [18]. This response seems to occur only in individuals who have asthma, because healthy subjects continue experiencing circadian fluctuations in airway caliber with nocturnal airway narrowing despite breathing air of constant temperature and humidity throughout the 24-hour period [19].

The role of exposure to allergens in bedding is a somewhat controversial issue. Some studies report nocturnal bronchoconstriction caused by experimental allergen inhalation (grain dust) [20], and reduction of circadian fluctuations in peak flow rates, frequency, and severity of asthma attacks through strict avoidance of allergens [21]. However, nocturnal bronchospasm occurs in both allergic and nonallergic asthma [22], and a study by Woodcock and colleagues [23] showed that allergen-impermeable bed covers for adults

who have asthma do not prevent nocturnal bronchoconstriction.

Gastroesophageal reflux disease (GERD) is commonly associated with nocturnal asthma symptoms. A cross-sectional study evaluated more than 2600 subjects, including more than 450 who had an existing diagnosis of asthma. Subjects who had GERD were significantly more likely to experience nighttime wheezing and breathlessness, and to report nocturnal cough and morning phlegm production than were subjects who did not have symptomatic GERD. Furthermore, physician-diagnosed asthma was twice as prevalent in subjects who had GERD (9%) compared with those who did not (4%), and peak flow variability was significantly greater in subjects who had symptomatic GERD [24]. In a study of different design, Cuttitta and colleagues [25] evaluated the relationship between GERD (manifested as reduced esophageal pH) and lower respiratory resistance. The most important predictor of change in lower respiratory resistance was the duration of esophageal acidosis. Collectively, these data suggest that GERD aggravates lower airway obstruction and worsens nocturnal asthma. Despite these compelling data linking the occurrence of GERD to symptoms of nocturnal asthma, proof is lacking showing that improvement in GERD translates to improvement in nocturnal asthma. A systematic literature review [26] of the effects of GERD treatment on asthma control found that neither medical therapy nor surgery for GERD was consistently related to improvement in asthma control.

Obesity is also associated with nocturnal asthma [24]. Hakala and colleagues [27] evaluated 14 obese patients who had asthma before and after significant weight loss. Diurnal and day-to-day variations in peak flow rates were significantly reduced by substantial weight loss, FEV_1 and midexpiratory flow rates increased, and airway resistance was reduced. Thus, obesity, per se, contributes to peak flow variability and diurnal variation in lung function. Whether weight loss reduced unrecognized GERD, OSA, or was an independent factor in improving lung function was not determined.

Snoring and OSA may cause worsening in asthma symptoms through an unknown mechanism. A study [28] on the role of snoring and OSA in nocturnal asthma showed that treatment of OSA with continuous positive airway pressure (CPAP) may be very helpful in alleviating asthma symptoms during sleep. Another study concluded that in some patients who have nocturnal asthma, OSA might be responsible for nocturnal symptoms. In this situation, CPAP improved nocturnal symptoms without amelioration in pulmonary function test abnormalities [29].

Mechanisms of nocturnal bronchoconstriction

Several mechanisms of nocturnal bronchial spasm have also been proposed, including circadian fluctuations in hormone levels, circadian variations in autonomic nervous systems' activity, airway inflammation, and genetic predisposition.

Hormones

The hormones of most interest in the study of nocturnal asthma are catecholamines, cortisol, and melatonin.

Catecholamines

Urinary adrenaline and noradrenalin excretion falls to a minimal level at night together with the lowest peak flow rates in patients who have asthma [30], but correction of the nocturnal fall of plasma adrenaline through adrenaline infusion does not eliminate nocturnal bronchoconstriction [31].

Cortisol

Nocturnal asthma symptoms were found to be most severe when the urinary excretion of 17-hydroxycorticosteroid was at its lowest and peak flow rates coincided with the highest levels of circulating steroids [22]. Treatment with large doses of steroids, however, did not prevent morning dipping [13]. A study in children who had asthma compared cortisol levels with FEV_1 measured every 4 hours and found that lower cortisol concentrations contributed to the presence of nocturnal airway obstruction in asthma [32]. A study by Sutherland and colleagues [33] measured plasma corticotropin and serum cortisol levels every 2 hours over a 24-hour period in patients who had nocturnal and nonnocturnal asthma and healthy control subjects. This study showed increased corticotropin levels in nocturnal asthma not accompanied by commensurate increase in cortisol levels, indicating blunted adrenal responsiveness in the nocturnal asthma phenotype.

Melatonin

Endogenous melatonin levels are elevated in individuals who have nocturnal asthma compared with those who have nonnocturnal asthma and healthy controls. This finding suggests that the elevated melatonin levels in nocturnal asthma might affect the severity of airway inflammation in this group [34]. Moreover, melatonin was shown to be proinflammatory in individuals who have asthma and healthy subjects. Patients who have nocturnal asthma showed the largest cytokine response [35], indicating differential immunomodulatory effects of melatonin, depending on the asthma phenotype.

Autonomic nervous system

The autonomic nervous system has three components: sympathetic, parasympathetic, and nonadrenergic–noncholinergic (NANC).

Bronchial muscles in humans have no direct sympathetic innervation. Bronchodilation is caused by catecholamines acting directly on bronchial smooth muscle. Diurnal fluctuations in β-adrenergic receptor sensitivity do not seem to contribute to nocturnal asthma. A study by Barnes and colleagues [36] showed that the bronchodilator effect of epinephrine was preserved during the night.

The parasympathetic system innervates bronchial muscle by way of the vagus nerve to produce bronchoconstriction. Parasympathetic activity is generally increased at night. Increased parasympathetic tone contributes significantly to the development of nocturnal asthma according to the results of studies using cholinergic blockade with atropine [37] and ipratropium [38].

The third component of the autonomic nervous system, the NANC, is the only known direct neural bronchodilating pathway in the human airway [39]. Its exact role and neurotransmitters are not well defined, but some evidence suggests that NANC activity level is at its nadir in the early morning [39], which may contribute to the tendency for increased bronchoconstriction and exaggerated asthma symptoms to occur during early hours.

Airway inflammation

Several studies have now confirmed that inflammation worsens in individuals who have nocturnal asthma during the nighttime hours, compared with those who have nonnocturnal asthma with comparable asthma severity. Parameters that increase at night include interleukin-1β [40], circulating eosinophils [41], bronchoalveolar lavage (BAL) eosinophils, and lymphocytes [42], and alveolar eosinophils, but not airway eosinophils [43]. In fact, studies showing no differences in inflammation are the exception [44,45].

The question that remains controversial, however, is why inflammation cycles have a diurnal rhythm. Most investigators view the circadian cycles of cortisol, cholinergic tone, histamine, and epinephrine as having theoretical relevance to inflammation, but the specific and detailed mechanistic links among these cycling biologic processes and the control of inflammation remain incompletely defined. Exhaled nitric oxide (eNO) has been suggested to be a noninvasive marker of airway inflammation. The accuracy of this assertion remains controversial. However, nitric oxide (NO) levels clearly increase in patients who have asthma compared with healthy controls, rise further after allergen challenge or asthma exacerbation, and fall with inhaled steroid therapy. Therefore evaluating eNO in the context of nocturnal asthma is an area of interest.

The literature is controversial regarding whether eNO levels and those of the synthetic enzyme responsible for the presence of most NO in exhaled breath, the inducible form of NO synthase (iNOS), rise and fall in circadian fashion. In a study of six patients who had asthma and experienced nocturnal symptoms, and eight who experienced no nocturnal symptoms, ten Hacken and colleagues [46] evaluated the variability of eNO in relationship to diurnal changes in airway function from 4:00 AM to 4:00 PM. Compared with healthy volunteers, the eNO level in patients who had asthma was higher. Among the patients who had asthma, those who experienced nocturnal symptoms showed increased eNO levels compared with those who had no nocturnal symptoms. Furthermore, a significant positive correlation occurred between circadian peak flow variability and eNO levels, suggesting that asthma severity was linked to increased eNO levels. However, no circadian variation of eNO was observed in any subject group (ie, healthy volunteers, subjects who had asthma without nocturnal symptoms, and subjects who had asthma with nocturnal symptoms).

Findings from a more recent study [47] of five patients who had nocturnal asthma and five patients who had asthma without nocturnal worsening were somewhat different from those in the study by ten Hacken and colleagues [46]. Patients who had nocturnal asthma had increased eNO levels compared with those who had asthma without nocturnal symptoms, but a circadian variation was observed only in those who had nocturnal asthma. The peak eNO level was achieved at 4:00 PM compared with 10:00 PM and 4:00 AM. Curiously, this peak corresponded to the time of best pulmonary function [47].

Perhaps in support of the findings of Georges and colleagues [47], ten Hacken and colleagues [48] quantitated iNOS expression in blood vessels in 25 patients who had asthma using bronchial biopsy. The expression of iNOS on blood vessels was greater in patients who had asthma than in controls. In a post hoc separation of patients who had asthma using the magnitude of peak expiratory flow (PEF) variability, those who had a PEF variability of more than 10% showed significantly greater expression of iNOS in blood vessels at 4:00 PM than at 4:00 AM. Thus, the same group has shown circadian variation in the levels of synthetic enzyme iNOS, but no variation in the levels of eNO. Clearly, the field of investigation of eNO is currently underdeveloped, and the implications of the observations remain somewhat obscure.

An intriguing area of research in nocturnal asthma is that of glucocorticoid resistance and signaling. Ongoing allergic inflammation can result in impaired function of the glucocorticoid receptor (GR). In this context, Kraft and colleagues [49] studied the binding affinity and function of the GR in patients who had asthma with nocturnal symptoms (n = 11) and without nocturnal symptoms (n = 12). Compared with healthy controls, patients who had asthma without nocturnal worsening showed significantly impaired glucocorticoid binding to GR. In patients who had nocturnal asthma, the abnormality was seen only at 4:00 AM, and GR binding was normal at 4:00 PM. This diurnal variation did not occur in the other groups. Functional data supported the biochemical analyses. The inhibition of lymphocyte proliferation through therapy with dexamethasone and hydrocortisone required an approximately 10-fold greater concentration of steroids at 4:00 AM than at 4:00 PM, suggesting a resistance to the effects of steroid therapy at 4:00 AM. The mechanisms through which these effects are mediated may include the increased expression GRβ, which is a splice variant of GR that binds corticosteroids but signals poorly [50]. In this follow-up study [50], GRβ expression was evaluated in patients who had asthma with and without nocturnal worsening. Patients who had nocturnal asthma showed increased expression of GRβ compared with those who had nonnocturnal asthma, and diurnal variation was evident only in those who had nocturnal asthma, with further increased expression of GRβ at 4:00 AM compared with 4:00 PM.

Genetics

An intriguing area of investigation has been the identification of single-nucleotide polymorphisms in the coding region of the β-adrenoceptor gene, which result in amino acid changes in the extracellular, transmembrane, and intracellular portions of the resulting protein [51]. Of these, the substitution of glycine at position 16 for arginine has been studied in the context of nocturnal asthma. This polymorphism results in increased agonist-dependent down-regulation of β-receptor expression, and therefore is plausibly linked to asthma. In a seminal study by Turki and colleagues [52], the phenotype of nocturnal asthma was significantly linked to homozygosity for glycine 16. However, Ramsay and colleagues [53] were unable to show a linkage between the glycine 16 polymorphism and any asthma phenotype. The variance in the study by Turki and colleagues [52] is likely the result of different genetic backgrounds among the patients studied, and highlights the difficulty in identifying specific genetic causes for complex diseases such as asthma. The role of other β-receptor polymorphisms, and particularly their interactions, requires additional study of large groups of well-characterized patients who have asthma.

Symptoms and signs

The essential features of sleep-related asthma are dyspnea, wheezing, coughing, air hunger, or chest tightness during sleep. These symptoms usually improve when bronchodilating medications are administered [54]. Sleep disruption and daytime sleepiness are the major presenting symptoms in individuals who have nocturnal asthma. They complain of dyspnea and wheezing that disrupt their sleep and cause daytime sleepiness and fatigue. Sleep disruption and daytime sleepiness have been verified with electroencephalogram [14,55] and neurocognitive studies [55]. Moreover, impairment of daytime cognitive function does not seem to be caused by pharmacotherapy side effects. If anything, successful asthma control with drug therapy has been shown to enhance cognitive function [8].

Death is fortunately an uncommon presentation of nocturnal asthma, but more individuals who have asthma die per hour of the night than per hour of the day [56]. The mortality rate in the general population is also higher during the night, but the average rate increase between midnight and 8:00 AM is only 5%, in contrast to the 28% death rate increase seen in patients who have asthma [57]. Increased death rate at night could be caused by several factors, including the inability of individuals who have asthma to be promptly awakened by hypoxia [57], hypercapnia [58], or increased airflow resistance [59], resulting in delayed medical help and treatment. Delay in home-based medical treatment secondary to lack of medical personnel does not seem to be a major contributor, however, because even in the hospital setting, most respiratory arrests occur in the early morning hours. Hetzel and colleagues [60] reported that most ventilatory arrests of hospitalized patients who have asthma occurred in the early morning. Nocturnal bronchospasm seems to be one of the most important causes of nocturnal death. In a prospective study, Bateman and Clarke [61] found that the two patients who had asthma who died at night had a pattern of wide diurnal fluctuations in PEFR.

Diagnosis

The diagnosis of sleep-related asthma requires the presence of asthma-related symptoms, including shortness of breath, wheezing, and cough occurring during the main sleep period (usually, but not invariably, at night) and is associated with a more than 15% decrement in overnight peak airflow rate.

Treatment of sleep-related asthma

According to current United States guidelines [10], nocturnal symptoms of asthma occurring more often than once weekly may indicate inadequate control of asthma. Because most patients who have nocturnal asthma have symptoms at least this frequently, most patients who have nocturnal asthma have persistent asthma of moderate or severe levels of severity, as determined by the guidelines. Furthermore, the preferred treatment for persistent asthma of these levels of severity is inhaled corticosteroids. Thus, most patients who have clinically important nocturnal asthma should probably be treated with an inhaled steroid as the primary controller agent. Many industry-sponsored clinical trials of controller medications (eg, inhaled steroids, leukotriene modifiers, long-acting β agonists, theophylline) have used nighttime symptoms as an index of efficacy. Without reviewing those trials in detail, each of these strategies can clearly reduce nighttime symptoms, and most can improve morning peak flow rates or FEV_1. These data suggest that controlling the underlying processes of asthma subsequently leads to improvements in nocturnal asthma. However, this information is subtly, but importantly, different from that of a focused investigation of nocturnal asthma in which all subjects have been selected for the presence of significant nighttime physiologic embarrassment. Theophylline has long been regarded as an important therapeutic tool in managing nocturnal asthma, because it can improve pulmonary function for a 12-hour period, particularly when administered in the evening. Moreover, theophylline reduces late-phase physiologic responses after allergen challenge and increases the tolerated dose of allergen in an experimental model [62]. However, as newer approaches become available, the usefulness of theophylline therapy may become more limited.

Using a crossover design, Selby and colleagues [63] evaluated salmeterol and theophylline using psychometric and QOL outcomes. Improvements in pulmonary function (measured with PEF rate) and most psychometric indexes were equivalently improved with either therapy. However, therapy with salmeterol outperformed that with theophylline in terms of the number of awakenings and arousals, and in QOL measures [63]. In the same year, Kraft and colleagues [64] evaluated salmeterol therapy for treating nocturnal asthma in a double-blind, placebo-controlled trial. Salmeterol therapy improved the use of rescue therapy with albuterol and reduced the number of nocturnal awakenings, but, unsurprisingly, did not alter airway hyperresponsiveness or any bronchoscopic measure of inflammation. Finally, Wiegand and colleagues [65] studied the effects of theophylline and salmeterol in a placebo-controlled randomized trial. Outcomes included parameters of sleep, symptoms of asthma, and pulmonary function. Therapy with theophylline was equivalent to that with placebo in this trial, whereas therapy with salmeterol preserved pulmonary function during the night.

Chronotherapy

One of the greatest challenges in nocturnal asthma treatment has been the timing of the dose to optimize therapeutic drug effect during periods of nocturnal worsening. A study by Pincus and colleagues [66] compared the beneficial and systemic effects of 800 µg of inhaled triamcinolone once daily at 3:00 PM versus conventional 200 µg four-times-daily dosing. The results of this study indicated that the single daily administration of inhaled triamcinolone at 3:00 PM has no increased systemic effects and produces similar improvement in efficacy variables. These authors then conducted further studies on the chronotherapy of asthma, comparing the effects of once-daily dosing schedules (8:00 AM or 5:30 PM) with those of traditional four-times-daily dosing,. They concluded that a single dose of inhaled steroids at 5:30 PM produces efficacy similar to four-times-daily dosing and is superior to a single dose at 8:00 AM [67].

A double-blind placebo-controlled study [68] evaluated the effects of a 50-mg oral dose of prednisone given at 8:00 AM, 3:00 PM, or 8:00 PM on overnight spirometry, blood eosinophil counts, and bronchoalveolar lavage cytology in seven individuals who had asthma. A single prednisone dose at 3:00 PM resulted in a reduction in the overnight percentage decrease in FEV_1 and improvement in the FEV_1 measured at 4:00 AM. In contrast, neither the 8:00-AM nor the 8:00-PM prednisone dose resulted in overnight spirometric improvement. After the 3:00-PM prednisone dose, blood eosinophil counts were also significantly reduced at both 8:00 PM and 4:00 AM. Lastly, the 3:00-PM dosing resulted in pancellular reduction in bronchoalveolar lavage cytology. These data support the relevance of prednisone dose timing for altering the inflammatory milieu and spirometric decline in nocturnal asthma [68].

Chronopharmacologic strategy can also be used in theophylline treatment. Martin and colleagues [69] compared two different sustained-release theophylline preparations in patients who had nocturnal asthma: a once-daily 24-hour theophylline preparation at 7:00 PM versus twice-daily 12-hour theophylline preparation at 7:00 AM and 7:00 PM.

During the night, the serum theophylline concentration was significantly higher with the once-daily regimen, and the awakening FEV_1 value was also improved. The authors concluded that patients who have nocturnal asthma need to focus their treatment on the nocturnal portion of the circadian cycle, and that higher serum theophylline concentration during this critical period is beneficial without interfering with sleep quality [69].

Controversies in sleep-related asthma

A key and recurring question in the field of nocturnal asthma is whether patients who have nocturnal asthma simply have asthma that is more severe (with nocturnal symptoms being one indicator of severity) or have a qualitatively different disorder. Data exist on both sides of this question, and therefore a definitive answer is not currently available. The results of several studies have supported the concept that nocturnal asthma is simply asthma that is quantitatively more severe and is therefore more likely to be associated with increased variation in airway function and an increased frequency of nighttime symptoms. A study from the Netherlands was consistent with this concept. Healthy controls (n = 13), patients who had asthma with high PEF variability (ie, >15%; n = 10), and patients who had with moderate PEF variability (ie, ≤15%; n = 15) were evaluated using physiologic assessment, BAL, and bronchial biopsy. Patients who had asthma with high PEF variability had lower FEV_1, lower provocative concentration of methacholine causing a 20% decline in FEV_1, and lower concentration of adenosine monophosphate causing a 20% decline in FEV_1, all suggesting a greater degree of asthma severity [70]. Patients who had high PEF variability showed no differences in lymphocyte, mast cell, and eosinophil markers between 4:00 AM and 4:00 PM. However, these measures of inflammation were significantly greater in subjects who had high PEF variability than in those who had moderate variability, suggesting that nocturnal asthma was simply more severe asthma. In fact, this point of view has been clearly detailed [71].

The results of physiologic studies, which are detailed later, have also been equivocal. In a study by Desjardin and colleagues [72] of individuals who had asthma with and without nocturnal symptoms who were well-matched for FEV_1, pulmonary capillary blood volume changes were seen only in those who had nocturnal asthma. This study is uncommon in the literature, in that physiologically matched control subjects who did not have nocturnal symptoms were included, and a specific distinction could be seen between patients who had nocturnal asthma and those who did not. Studies by Irvin and colleagues [73] and Kraft and colleagues [74], although provocative, did not include FEV$_1$-matched controls who had asthma without nocturnal disease. Nocturnal and nonnocturnal asthma can be most clearly differentiated in the area of cellular and molecular indexes of inflammation. Diurnal variations in alveolar tissue inflammation, cytokine levels, and reactive oxygen species levels have been shown. However, many other studies have clearly shown that nocturnal asthma is associated with increased numbers of markers of inflammation, suggesting increased disease severity, but that the measured inflammatory markers do not cycle with circadian timing. Thus, although the literature does not currently distinguish between nocturnal asthma as a distinct entity and as a marker of severity, individuals who have more severe asthma clearly may also have a prominent nocturnal component to their disease. Understanding the mechanisms through which the master clock influences airway inflammation, airway function, and symptoms of asthma will undoubtedly lead to important insights into the pathogenesis of asthma.

Summary

Further research is needed to (1) elucidate the mechanisms of the coupling of central master clock signals to the regulation of inflammation and airway physiology; (2) distinguish the mechanisms that cause nighttime asthma from those that are a consequence of increased airway obstruction at night; (3) establish the most appropriate treatment strategy for nocturnal asthma symptoms, including effective treatment for GERD; and (4) match asthma populations with and without nocturnal worsening for FEV$_1$ or other markers of asthma severity to better understand the immunologic, inflammatory, and physiologic features that are most directly related to nighttime worsening of airway function.

References

[1] Braman SS. The global burden of asthma. Chest 2006;130(1 Suppl):4S–12S.

[2] Martin RJ. Location of airway inflammation in asthma and the relationship to circadian change in lung function. Chronobiol Int 1999;16:623–30.

[3] Turner-Warwick M. Epidemiology of nocturnal asthma. Am J Med 1988;85:6–8.

[4] Dethlefsen U, Repgas R. Ein neues Therapieprinzip bei Nachtlichen Asthma. Klin Med 1985;80:44–7.

[5] Raherison C, Abouelfath A, Le Gros V, et al. Underdiagnosis of nocturnal symptoms in asthma in general practice. J Asthma 2006;43(3):199–202.

[6] Calhoun WJ. Nocturnal asthma. Chest 2003;123:399S–405S.

[7] Diette GB, Markson L, Skinner EA, et al. Nocturnal asthma in children affects school attendance, school performance, and parents' work attendance. Arch Pediatr Adolesc Med 2000;154:923–8.

[8] Weersink EJM, van Zomeren EH, Koeter GH, et al. Treatment of nocturnal airway obstruction improves daytime cognitive performance in asthmatics. Am J Respir Crit Care Med 1997;156:1144–50.

[9] Stores G, Ellis AJ, Wiggs L, et al. Sleep and psychological disturbance in nocturnal asthma. Arch Dis Child 1998;78(5):413–9.

[10] National Asthma Education and Prevention Program. Expert panel report 2: guidelines for the diagnosis and prevention of asthma. Bethesda (MD): National Institutes of Health; April 1997. Publication No. 97–405.

[11] Sutherland ER. Nocturnal asthma. J Allergy Clin Immunol 2005;116(6):1179–86. [quiz: 1187; Epub 2005 Nov 8].

[12] Hetzel MR, Clark TJ. Does sleep cause nocturnal asthma? Thorax 1979;34:749–54.

[13] Clark TJ, Hetzel MR. Diurnal variation of asthma. Br J Dis Chest 1977;71:87–92.

[14] Kales A, Beall GN, Bajor GF, et al. Sleep studies in asthmatic adults: Relationship of attacks to sleep stage and time of night. J Allergy 1968;41:164–73.

[15] Martin RJ, Cicutto LC, Ballard RD. Factors related to the nocturnal worsening of asthma. Am Rev Respir Dis 1990;141:33–8.

[16] Hendeles L, Beaty R, Ahrens R, et al. Response to inhaled albuterol during nocturnal asthma. J Allergy Clin Immunol 2004;113:1058–62.

[17] Whyte KF, Douglas NJ. Posture and nocturnal asthma. Thorax 1989;44:579–81.

[18] Chen WY, Chai H. Airway cooling and nocturnal asthma. Chest 1982;81:675–80.

[19] Kerr HD. Diurnal variation of respiratory function independent of air quality: experience with an environmentally controlled exposure chamber for human subjects. Arch Environ Health 1973;26:144–52.

[20] Davies RJ, Green M, Schofield NM. Recurrent nocturnal asthma after exposure to grain dust. Am Rev Respir Dis 1976;114:1011–9.

[21] Platts-Mills TA, Tovey ER, Mitchell EB, et al. Reduction of bronchial hyperreactivity during prolonged allergen avoidance. Lancet 1982;2:675–8.

[22] Connolly CK. Diurnal rhythms in airway obstruction. Br J Dis Chest 1979;73:357–66.

[23] Woodcock A, Forster L, Matthews E, et al. Control of exposure to mite allergen and allergen-impermeable bed covers for adults with asthma. N Engl J Med 2003;349:225–36.

[24] Gislason T, Janson C, Vermeire P, et al. Respiratory symptoms and nocturnal gastroesophageal reflux. Chest 2002;121:158–63.

[25] Cuttitta G, Cibella F, Visconti A, et al. Spontaneous gastroesophageal reflux and airway patency during the night in adult asthmatics. Am J Respir Crit Care Med 2000;161:177–81.

[26] Coughlan JL, Gibson PG, Henry RL. Medical treatment for reflux oesophagitis does not consistently improve asthma control: a systematic review. Thorax 2000;56:198–204.

[27] Hakala K, Stenius-Aarniala B, Sovijarvi A. Effects of weight loss on peak flow variability, airways obstruction, and lung volumes in obese patients with asthma. Chest 2000;118:1315–21.

[28] Chan CS, Woolcock AJ, Sullivan CE. Nocturnal asthma: role of snoring and obstructive sleep apnea. Am Rev Respir Dis 1988;137:1502–4.

[29] Ciftci TU, Ciftci B, Guven SF, et al. Effect of nasal continuous positive airway pressure in uncontrolled nocturnal asthmatic patients with obstructive sleep apnea syndrome. Respir Med 2005;99(5):529–34. [Epub 2004 Nov 23].

[30] Soutar CA, Carruthers M, Pickering CA. Nocturnal asthma and urinary adrenaline and noradrenaline excretion. Thorax 1977;32:677–83.

[31] Morrison JF, Teale C, Pearson SB, et al. Adrenaline and nocturnal asthma. BMJ 1990;301:473–6.

[32] Landstra AM, Postma DS, Boezen HM, et al. Role of serum cortisol levels in children with asthma. Am J Respir Crit Care Med 2002;165:708–12.

[33] Sutherland ER, Ellison MC, Kraft M, et al. Altered pituitary-adrenal interaction in nocturnal asthma. J Allergy Clin Immunol 2003;112:52–7.

[34] Sutherland ER, Ellison MC, Kraft M, et al. Elevated serum melatonin is associated with the nocturnal worsening of asthma. J Allergy Clin Immunol 2003;112:513–7.

[35] Sutherland ER, Martin RJ, Ellison MC, et al. Immunomodulatory effects of melatonin in asthma. Am J Respir Crit Care Med 2002;166:1055–61.

[36] Barnes P, FitzGerald G, Brown M, et al. Nocturnal asthma and changes in circulating epinephrine, histamine, and cortisol. N Engl J Med 1980;303:263–7.

[37] Morrison JF, Pearson SB, Dean HG. Parasympathetic nervous system in nocturnal asthma. Br Med J (Clin Res Ed) 1988;296:1427–9.

[38] Catterall JR, Rhind GB, Whyte KF, et al. Is nocturnal asthma caused by changes in airway cholinergic activity? Thorax 1988;43:720–4.

[39] Mackay TW, Hulks G, Douglas NJ. Non-adrenergic, non-cholinergic function in the human airway. Respir Med 1998;92:461–6.

[40] Jarjour NN, Busse WW. Cytokines in bronchoalveolar lavage fluid of patients with nocturnal asthma. Am J Respir Crit Care Med 1995;152:1474–7.

[41] Bates ME, Clayton M, Calhoun W, et al. Relationship of plasma epinephrine and circulating eosinophils to nocturnal asthma. Am J Respir Crit Care Med 1994;149:667–72.

[42] Mackay TW, Wallace WAH, Howie SEM, et al. Role of inflammation in nocturnal asthma. Thorax 1994;49:257–62.

[43] Kraft M, Djukanovic R, Wilson S, et al. Alveolar tissue inflammation in asthma. Am J Respir Crit Care Med 1996;154:1505–10.

[44] Postma DS, Oosterhoff Y, Van Aalderen WMC, et al. Inflammation in nocturnal asthma? Am J Respir Crit Care Med 1994;150:S83–6.

[45] Oosterhoff Y, Hoogsteden HC, Rutgers B, et al. Lymphocyte and macrophage activation in bronchoalveolar lavage fluid in nocturnal asthma. Am J Respir Crit Care Med 1995;151:75–81.

[46] ten Hacken NHT, van der Vaart H, van der Mark TW, et al. Exhaled nitric oxide is higher both at day and night in subjects with nocturnal asthma. Am J Respir Crit Care Med 1998;158:902–7.

[47] Georges G, Bartelson BB, Martin RJ, et al. Circadian variation in exhaled nitric oxide in nocturnal asthma. J Asthma 1999;36:467–73.

[48] ten Hacken NH, Postma DS, Drok G, et al. Increased vascular expression of iNOS at day but not at night in asthmatic subjects with increased nocturnal airway obstruction. Eur Respir J 2000;16:445–51.

[49] Kraft M, Vianna E, Martin RJ, et al. Nocturnal asthma is associated with reduced glucocorticoid receptor binding affinity and decreased steroid responsiveness at night. J Allergy Clin Immunol 1999;103:66–71.

[50] Kraft M, Hamid Q, Chrousos GP, et al. Decreased steroid responsiveness at night in nocturnal asthma: is the macrophage responsible? Am J Respir Crit Care Med 2001;163:1219–25.

[51] Liggett SB. Polymorphisms of the beta 2-adrenergic receptor and asthma. Am J Respir Crit Care Med 1997;156:S156–62.

[52] Turki J, Pak J, Green SA, et al. Genetic polymorphisms of the beta 2-adrenergic receptor in nocturnal and nonnocturnal asthma: evidence that Gly16 correlates with the nocturnal phenotype. J Clin Invest 1995;95:1635–41.

[53] Ramsay CE, Hayden CM, Tiller KJ, et al. Polymorphisms in the beta2-adrenoreceptor gene are associated with decreased airway responsiveness. Clin Exp Allergy 1999;29:1195–203.

[54] American Academy of Sleep Medicine. International classification of sleep disorders, revised: diagnostic and coding manual. Rochester (MN); 2001.

[55] Fitzpatrick MF, Engleman H, Whyte KF, et al. Morbidity in nocturnal asthma: sleep quality and daytime cognitive performance. Thorax 1991;46:569–73.

[56] Douglas NJ. Asthma at night. Clin Chest Med 1985;6:663–74.

[57] Douglas NJ, White DP, Weil JV, et al. Hypoxic ventilatory response decreases during sleep in

normal men. Am Rev Respir Dis 1982;125: 286–9.

[58] Douglas NJ, White DP, Weil JV, et al. Hypercapnic ventilatory response in sleeping adults. Am Rev Respir Dis 1982;126:758–62.

[59] Gugger M, Molloy J, Gould GA, et al. Ventilatory and arousal responses to added inspiratory resistance during sleep. Am Rev Respir Dis 1989;140: 1301–7.

[60] Hetzel MR, Clark TJ, Branthwaite MA. Asthma: analysis of sudden deaths and ventilatory arrests in hospital. BMJ 1977;1:808–11.

[61] Bateman JR, Clarke SW. Sudden death in asthma. Thorax 1979;34:40–4.

[62] Jarjour NN, Lacouture PG, Busse WW. Theophylline inhibits the late asthmatic response to nighttime antigen challenge in patients with mild atopic asthma. Ann Allergy Asthma Immunol 1998;81:231–6.

[63] Selby C, Engleman HM, Fitzpatrick MF, et al. Inhaled salmeterol or oral theophylline in nocturnal asthma? Am J Respir Crit Care Med 1997; 155:104–8.

[64] Kraft M, Wenzel SE, Bettinger CM, et al. The effect of salmeterol on nocturnal symptoms, airway function, and inflammation in asthma. Chest 1997;111:1249–54.

[65] Wiegand L, Mende CN, Zaidel G, et al. Salmeterol vs theophylline: sleep and efficacy outcomes in patients with nocturnal asthma. Chest 1999; 115:1525–32.

[66] Pincus DJ, Szefler SJ, Ackerson LM, et al. Chronotherapy of asthma with inhaled steroids: the effect of dosage timing on drug efficacy. J Allergy Clin Immunol 1995;95:1172–8.

[67] Pincus DJ, Humeston TR, Martin RJ. Further studies on the chronotherapy of asthma with inhaled steroids: the effect of dosage timing on drug efficacy. J Allergy Clin Immunol 1997;100: 771–4.

[68] Beam WR, Weiner DE, Martin RJ. Timing of prednisone and alterations of airways inflammation in nocturnal asthma. Am Rev Respir Dis 1992;146:1524–30.

[69] Martin RJ, Cicutto LC, Ballard RD, et al. Circadian variations in theophylline concentrations and the treatment of nocturnal asthma. Am Rev Respir Dis 1989;139:475–8.

[70] ten Hacken NHT, Timens W, Smith M, et al. Increased peak expiratory flow variation in asthma: severe persistent increased but not nocturnal worsening of airway inflammation. Eur Respir J 1998;12:546–50.

[71] Weersink EJM, Postma DS. Nocturnal asthma: not a separate disease entity. Respir Med 1994; 88:483–91.

[72] Desjardin JA, Sutrarik JM, Suh BY, et al. Influence of sleep on pulmonary capillary volume in normal and asthmatic subjects. Am J Respir Crit Care Med 1995;152:193–8.

[73] Irvin CG, Pak J, Martin RJ. Airway-parenchyma uncoupling in nocturnal asthma. Am J Respir Crit Care Med 2000;161:50–6.

[74] Kraft M, Pak J, Martin RJ, et al. Distal lung dysfunction at night in nocturnal asthma. Am J Respir Crit Care Med 2001;163:1551–6.

SLEEP
MEDICINE
CLINICS

Sleep Med Clin 2 (2007) 19–29

Sleep and Glucose Intolerance/Diabetes Mellitus

Mary Ip, MD[a],*, Babak Mokhlesi, MD, MSc[b]

Glucose metabolism and its clinical disorders

Diabetes mellitus is a group of metabolic disorders characterized by chronic hyperglycemia caused by various pathogenetic processes in glucose homeostasis [1,2]. In health, glucose homeostasis is achieved by regulating glucose production by the liver (gluconeogenesis) and glucose use by insulin-dependent tissues, such as muscle and fat, and non–insulin-dependent tissues, such as the brain [3]. Insulin is secreted by pancreatic β cells, both constitutionally and acutely in response to glucose loading, and its vital function is to mediate glucose disposal by peripheral tissues. It also suppresses hepatic gluconeogenesis and adipose tissue lipolysis. The biologic response of target tissues to the actions of insulin (insulin sensitivity) has many physiologic determinants, the major one being adiposity (Box 1), and impairment of tissue response (insulin resistance) results in reduced glucose disposal [4].

Insulin resistance plays a major role in the development of type 2 diabetes [5] and some other disease states (Box 1).

Two major forms of diabetes mellitus exist. Type 1 diabetes is caused primarily by β-cell destruction that results in insulin deficiency, whereas type 2 diabetes, which is the most prevalent form, is characterized by insulin resistance with relative deficient insulin secretion (inadequate compensatory hyperinsulinemia), although some individuals may have predominant insulin deficiency. Both genetics and environmental factors are important in the pathogenesis of type 2 diabetes, and abdominal obesity is an important risk factor.

Clinically, diabetes mellitus has stages of disease progression [1,6]. Impaired glucose regulation is the intermediate stage between normal glucose tolerance and diabetes, and can be identified by impaired fasting glucose or impaired glucose tolerance, which is assessed with an oral glucose tolerance test. This metabolic state is predictive of type 2 diabetes.

[a] Division of Respiratory and Critical Care Medicine, University Department of Medicine, 4th Floor, Professorial Block, Queen Mary Hospital, Pokfulam, Hong Kong, China
[b] Section of Pulmonary and Critical Care, Sleep Disorders Center, The University of Chicago Pritzker School of Medicine, 5841 South Maryland Avenue, MC 0999/Room L11B, Chicago, IL 60637, USA
* Corresponding author.
E-mail address: msmip@hkucc.hku.hk (M. Ip).

doi:10.1016/j.jsmc.2006.12.002

Box 1:   Determinants of insulin sensitivity

Well-established determinants
Adiposity
Diet
Exercise and physical activity
Stress
Hyperglycemia

Possible determinants
Sleep, sleep deprivation, and sleep-related disorders

Insulin resistance or glucose intolerance is also an intrinsic component of the metabolic syndrome (insulin resistance syndrome) [7,8], which is a cluster of cardiometabolic risk factors. Although different sets of defining criteria have been proposed for this syndrome, most experts agree that these consist of insulin resistance and glucose intolerance, abdominal obesity, hypertension, and dyslipidemia (hypertriglyceridemia and low high-density lipoprotein cholesterol) [9,10]. Other features that are related include hyperuricemia, inflammatory and thrombogenic profile, hyperleptinemia, and microalbuminuria [8,11].

Diabetes mellitus carries major morbidity and is among the five leading causes of death from disease in many countries [12], attributed to its devastating complications, particularly cardiovascular disease. Moreover, as obesity becomes epidemic, the prevalence of diabetes will also rise [13]. Type 2 diabetes afflicted an estimated 5% of the world's population in 2003. In the United States, its prevalence is estimated to rise from 14.2% in 2003 to 26.2% in 2025, and the rise is forecasted to be particularly sharp in Asia [14].

Sleep and glucose metabolism

Influence of sleep on glucose metabolism

Contrary to most mammals, human sleep is generally consolidated into a single 7- to 9-hour period,

---

Box 2:   Common clinical states associated with insulin resistance

Type 2 diabetes mellitus
Metabolic syndrome
Hypertension
Polycystic ovary syndrome
Nonalcoholic fatty liver disease
Obstructive sleep apnea
Insulin resistance as a secondary phenomenon in:
    Acute illness
    Cushing's syndrome
    Pregnancy

---

leading to an extended period of fasting overnight. Both pancreatic β-cell responsiveness and insulin sensitivity are influenced by sleep. Despite the extended fast during overnight sleep, blood glucose levels remain stable or fall only minimally. By comparison, when individuals are awake and fasting in a recumbent position without any physical activity, glucose levels decrease an average of 10 to 20 mg/dL over a 12-hour period [15].

Therefore, several mechanisms operative during nocturnal sleep must intervene to maintain stable glucose levels during the overnight fast. Sleep and the circadian rhythm play roles in modulating insulin production, insulin sensitivity, glucose use, and thus glucose tolerance throughout the night. In normal healthy individuals, glucose tolerance varies throughout the day; plasma glucose responses to exogenous glucose are markedly higher in the evening than in the morning, and glucose tolerance is at its minimum in the middle of the night [15]. The reduced glucose tolerance during the evening and sleep is partly caused by a reduction in insulin sensitivity concomitant with a reduction in the insulin secretory response, a marked reduction in cerebral glucose uptake because of slow-wave sleep, and a reduction in peripheral glucose use [16,17]. During the latter part of the night, glucose tolerance begins to improve, and glucose levels progressively decrease toward morning values, reflecting increased glucose uptake partly because of decreased slow-wave sleep and increased rapid eye movement sleep. These major modulatory effects of sleep on glucose regulation can also be observed when the sleep period occurs during the daytime [18].

Sleep duration or sleep disturbance and glucose homeostasis

Duration of sleep is essentially determined by individual and societal behavioral modes. Voluntary sleep curtailment to the minimum tolerable duration is highly prevalent and has become a hallmark of the modern society. Surveys conducted by the National Sleep Foundation [19] in the United States have documented that self-reported sleep duration of Americans has decreased by 1.5 to 2 hours over the past 40 years. The proportion of young adults reporting that they sleep less than 7 hours per night increased from 16% in 1960 to 37% in 2002 [20]. More than 30% of middle-aged men and women report sleeping less than 6 hours per night [21]. The dramatic increase in the incidence of obesity and diabetes over the past 3 to 4 decades [22] overlaps the progressive decrease in self-reported sleep duration.

Because sleep itself modulates glucose tolerance and homeostasis, changes in the quantity or quality of sleep may affect glucose tolerance. Voluntary sleep curtailment can cause decreased sleep quantity, whereas chronic intrinsic sleep disorders such as insomnia or sleep-disordered breathing (SDB) can affect both sleep quality and quantity. Both conditions are highly prevalent in the community. Chronic insomnia occurs in 6% to 15% of the general adult population [23]. In middle-aged adults, SDB (apnea–hypopnea index [AHI] ≥5) has been reported to affect 24% of men and 9% of women [24]. This article reviews the growing body of experimental and epidemiologic evidence linking sleep loss and sleep disturbance with alterations in glucose homeostasis.

Laboratory studies on sleep and glucose metabolism

Although initial animal studies that subjected rats to prolonged total sleep deprivation were unable to show elevated fasting glucose levels despite a marked increase in food intake by the rodents [25,26], total sleep deprivation in humans resulted in decreased glucose tolerance or increased food intake [27]. However, in daily life, partial sleep deprivation, either acute or chronic, is more common than total sleep deprivation. A landmark study evaluating the effect of short-term partial sleep deprivation on glucose homeostasis subjected 11 young, healthy, lean men to sleep restriction of 4 hours per night over 6 days followed by 7 days of sleep extension of 12 hours per night. After 6 days of sleep restriction, evidence of impaired glucose tolerance was seen. Furthermore, with sleep restriction, the mean leptin level—an anorexigenic hormone produced by adipocytes—was 19% lower and sympathetic nervous system activity was increased [28]. The degree of decrease in the acute insulin response with short-term sleep curtailment was similar to that observed in aging and gestational diabetes [29,30].

The same investigators repeated the experiment in 12 healthy men, but used a randomized crossover design. In this study, the sleep curtailment was limited to 2 days. Despite a shorter manipulation of sleep duration, evidence of impaired glucose tolerance was still seen. When compared with extended sleep, 2 days of sleep curtailment led to higher glucose levels, lower insulin levels, and a 30% increase in appetite for high caloric density carbohydrates. The anorexigenic hormone leptin decreased by 18% and levels of the orexigenic factor ghrelin—a stomach-derived peptide that stimulates appetite—increased by 28%, matching the significant increase in hunger and appetite on a visual analog scale [31].

Mechanistic links mediating the effects of sleep loss on glucose homeostasis

The mechanisms behind alterations in glucose homeostasis after recurrent partial sleep restriction are multifactorial (Box 3). In addition to a decrease in cerebral glucose metabolism, a reduction in insulin release occurs, probably because of increased sympathetic nervous activity at the level of the pancreatic β cell. Furthermore, alterations in the secretory profiles of the counter-regulatory hormones may also contribute to the disturbances of glucose homeostasis, causing elevated nighttime growth hormone and evening cortisol levels [15,32,33]. Proinflammatory cytokines can increase with even 1 night of partial sleep loss [34]. A low-grade inflammation caused by chronic sleep loss may predispose to insulin resistance and diabetes [35,36].

Taken together, these laboratory studies suggest that sleep loss and sleep disturbances contribute to the development of insulin resistance and type 2 diabetes through multiple pathways, including a deleterious effect on glucose homeostasis, increased inflammation, and adversely affecting appetite regulation, leading to increased food intake, weight gain, and ultimately obesity (Box 3) [37].

Observational and epidemiologic studies on sleep duration and disturbance, and glucose intolerance and diabetes mellitus

Several population-based or large cohort studies have examined the relationship between the amount or quality of sleep and glucose tolerance [38–50].

The Sleep Heart Health Study (SHHS) data showed that sleep duration of either 6 hours or less or 9 hours or more was associated with increased prevalence of diabetes or glucose intolerance, compared with 7 to 8 hours of sleep per night, adjusted for AHI and other confounders [38]. The Nurses Health study included approximately 70,000 middle-aged women who did not

---

Box 3: Mechanisms linking sleep and sleep loss to altered glucose homeostasis

Sleep
Reduced insulin sensitivity
Reduced insulin secretory response to elevated glucose level
Decrease cerebral glucose use related to slow-wave sleep
Reduction in peripheral glucose use

Sleep loss
Impaired glucose tolerance
Increased appetite and hunger (elevation of ghrelin and reduction of leptin)
Increased sympathetic nervous system activity
Alterations in counter-regulatory hormones (growth hormone and cortisol)
Increased proinflammatory markers

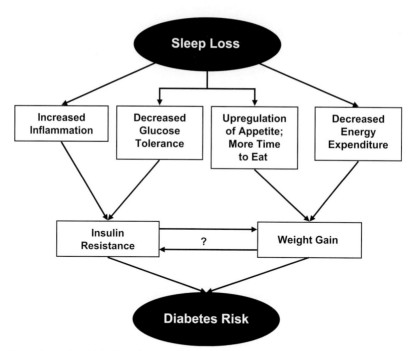

Fig. 1. Mechanisms through which sleep loss may lead to weight gain and increased risk for type 2 diabetes. (*Adapted from* Knutson K, Spiegel K, Penev P, et al. Metabolic consequences of sleep deprivation. Sleep Med Rev, in press; with permission.)

have diabetes mellitus at baseline, and showed that both short and long sleepers had significantly increased risks for developing diabetes after 10 years, although the risk became nonsignificant in the short sleepers after adjustment for body mass index (BMI) and other confounders [39]. For the 1187 subjects who had symptomatic diabetes, the adjusted risk ratios were modestly elevated in both short and long sleepers. In more than 1100 men in the Massachusetts Male Aging Study, those reporting shorter and longer sleep duration were two and three times as likely to develop incident diabetes, respectively [40]. In two Swedish studies, men, but not women, who experienced shorter duration of sleep were found to have increased incident diabetes in a 12-year follow-up. Similarly, no association between sleep duration at baseline and diabetic risk was shown in women in a 32-year follow-up [41,42].

The influence of sleep quality on glucose tolerance has also been investigated in several longitudinal cohorts [41–45]. All except one study [42] reported an increased risk for incident diabetes in relation to sleep disturbances, such as difficulty initiating sleep, difficulty maintaining sleep, need for regular use of hypnotics, or frequently disrupted sleep.

In addition to studies of the general population, several studies evaluated sleep duration or sleep quality in individuals who have diabetes mellitus [46–50]. Most found that poor sleep quality was more prevalent in individuals who had diabetes compared with those who did not [46,48–50], and that this adversely influenced diabetic control [49,50].

An increase in obesity will also pose increased risk for glucose intolerance, and studies have addressed the issue of sleep and obesity. Studies in Japanese adults and children and the United States adult primary care population have shown that sleeping less increased the likelihood of obesity [51–54]. Data from 1024 subjects in the Wisconsin Sleep Cohort Study showed that 5 hours of habitual sleep compared with 8 hours led to hormonal changes promoting appetite, independent of SDB and other confounding factors. Furthermore, the increase in BMI was proportional to the decrease in sleep duration [54]. The degree of hormonal changes promoting appetite in this study was strikingly comparable to a previously reported laboratory study of partial sleep restriction [31].

Taken together, the findings of observational and epidemiologic studies validate those of the laboratory studies: that sleep disturbance can lead to alterations in glucose homeostasis, adversely affect appetite and hunger, and ultimately increase the risk for obesity and type 2 diabetes.

Sleep-disordered breathing and glucose metabolism

Obstructive sleep apnea (OSA) is the most common form of SDB worldwide [55,56]. A high association between OSA and glucose intolerance/diabetes mellitus would not be unexpected because they share the common risk factor of obesity. Research momentum has focused on the hunt for evidence of independent pathogenetic links between SDB and glucose metabolism disorders. The identification of a causal role would have implications not only on the understanding of disease pathogenesis but also on clinical management. The spreading obesity epidemic and the high prevalence of OSA and diabetes mellitus pose a colossal threat to health care [57].

Relationship between sleep-disordered breathing and derangements in glucose metabolism

Several epidemiologic studies consistently showed that heavy snoring with or without observed breathing pauses was associated with increased frequency of disturbances of glucose metabolism, independent of obesity [58–63].

In a population-based sample of 116 men who had hypertension, 25 had diabetes mellitus. Although obesity was the main risk factor for diabetes, coexistent severe OSA added to the risk, and SDB influenced plasma insulin and glycemia independently of central obesity [63]. In 150 healthy, overweight, middle-aged men recruited from the community, OSA (defined as AHI ≥ 5) was associated with a twofold risk for glucose intolerance, independent of BMI and percent body fat measured with hydrodensitometry [64]. The impairment in glucose tolerance correlated with the severity of oxygen desaturation, whereas an increasing AHI was independently associated with worsening insulin resistance.

Among 2656 participants of the SHHS, those who had mild or moderate-to-severe OSA based on AHI criteria had increased risks (risk ratios of 1.27 and 1.46, respectively) for fasting glucose intolerance [65]. Sleep-related hypoxemia was associated with glucose intolerance independent of age, gender, BMI, and waist circumference.

Subjects in the SHHS who had diabetes mellitus were reported to experience more periodic breathing and central apneas than obstructive events [66]. Only periodic breathing was significantly and independently associated with diabetes when adjusted for confounders, and the breathing disorder was attributed to autonomic dysfunction. This finding contrasts with that reported by many other studies, population-based or clinic-based, in which a high association was seen between obstructive, rather than central, sleep apnea and diabetes mellitus.

The relationship between SDB and metabolic dysfunction has been investigated repeatedly in subjects recruited from clinical settings [67,68]. Findings involving smaller sample sizes conflict, with some showing a positive independent relationship [69,70], whereas others do not [71,72]. Studies with larger sample sizes have more consistently reported a positive independent association between SDB and insulin resistance/glucose intolerance [73–75] or the metabolic syndrome [76,77]. In a clinic sample of 261 subjects, the severity of SDB was associated with higher fasting insulin, but not glucose, with adjustment for BMI [73]. In 270 Chinese subjects who had polysomnograms in the sleep laboratory, insulin resistance, indicated by the homeostasis model assessment of fasting insulin and glucose measurements, was independently predicted by obesity and, to a lesser extent, AHI, and insulin resistance was a determinant of hypertension [74]. In a case-controlled study, whole-body and hepatic insulin sensitivity indices were significantly lower in individuals who had OSA compared with obese controls who did not have OSA and normal-weight controls, with adjustment for obesity and age, whereas insulin secretion was similar in the three groups [75].

Recently, a study in the United Kingdom assessed the risk for OSA in 1682 men who had type 2 diabetes using a survey followed by overnight oximetry in 240 men selected from groups considered to be at high or low risk for OSA. The study found that approximately 23% of the men who had type 2 diabetes had OSA [78], and that OSA was significantly associated with diabetes mellitus ($P = .03$), independent of BMI and neck circumference.

Data on children are scanty. One study of obese children showed significant correlations between AHI and fasting insulin independent of BMI [79]. However, two subsequent studies reported that insulin resistance was related to BMI rather than severity of SDB [80,81].

Several prospective population-cohorts have evaluated for new incident diabetes on longitudinal assessment. In Sweden and the United States, middle-aged men and women, respectively, have been followed-up for 10 years or more, and snoring at baseline was found to be associated with increased incident diabetes [82,83]. However, in an analysis of the Wisconsin Sleep Study Cohort

[84], despite an independent association between SDB and insulin resistance at baseline, new incidence of diabetes over 4 years' follow-up was not more in subjects who had a baseline AHI of 5 or more compared with those who had an AHI less than 5.

Treatment intervention studies

In contrast to epidemiologic or observational studies, treatment intervention studies have been much less positive regarding the pathogenic role of OSA [67], and most failed to show any improvement in glucose metabolism [71,85–92].

More recently, several studies reported a positive treatment effect of OSA on insulin resistance or diabetic control. Using the hyperinsulinemic euglycemic clamp in 40 men who had severe OSA, 2 nights of treatment with continuous positive airway pressure (CPAP) led to significant improvement in insulin sensitivity, and the effect was sustained after 3 months of therapy. The improvement in insulin sensitivity was more marked in patients who were not obese compared with those who were [93]. Another study evaluated glycemic control with HbA1c and interstitial glucose levels using a continuous glucose monitoring system in 25 patients who had diabetes and OSA [94]. Treatment of OSA with CPAP reduced morning postprandial glucose values, and those who had worse initial glycemic control showed a significant decrease in HbA1c. A retrospective cohort analysis of 38 subjects who had diabetes and severe OSA similarly showed that HbA1c decreased after CPAP treatment for several months [95]. In one study, a population-based sample of 38 men who had severe OSA treated with CPAP for 3 weeks showed a decrease in insulin resistance and increase in insulin-like growth factor-1 (IGF-1) compared with controls who had an AHI less than 10 and did not undergo treatment [96].

Although the data from these recent intervention studies are encouraging, preliminary data from a randomized controlled study of therapeutic CPAP versus sham-CPAP reported that neither insulin resistance, evaluated with euglycemic clamp studies, nor diabetic control, indicated by HbA1c, showed any significant change with treatment of OSA [97].

Mechanistic links of sleep-disordered breathing and derangements of glucose metabolism

In line with the mediation of the effect of sleep on glucose metabolism, the mechanistic links of SDB and regulation of glucose metabolism are likely multifaceted (Fig. 2) [98]. The common factor of

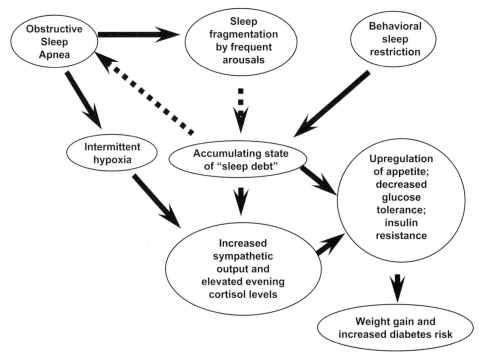

Fig. 2. Putative mechanisms leading to insulin resistance and increased diabetes risk in obstructive sleep apnea. (*Adapted from* Spiegel K, Knutson K, Leproult R, et al. Sleep loss: a novel risk factor for insulin resistance and type 2 diabetes. J Appl Physiol 2005;99:2008–19.)

adiposity cannot be ignored, but both theoretical basis and evidence suggest that SDB itself may generate pathogenetic effects on glucose homeostasis.

OSA is believed to pose chronic stress caused by recurrent intermittent hypoxia and cerebral arousals. The recurrent sleep fragmentation and disrupted sleep architecture also cause sleep loss. These adverse physiologic effects may trigger downstream mechanisms that promote insulin resistance or glucose intolerance.

The role of counter-regulatory hormones of glucose metabolism have been investigated in OSA. Enhanced sympathetic activity has been shown consistently in OSA, reflected by microneurography of skeletal muscles [99] or increased catecholamines in plasma or urine [100,101] that improved with effective control of OSA. Several studies showed that the magnitude of sympathetic activation correlated with the severity of hypoxemia in OSA [102,103].

Other aspects of hypothalamic–pituitary–adrenal axis activation have been more controversial. The timing of measurements may be an important factor, because hormones have intrinsic diurnal rhythms and spot measurements may not be sufficiently sensitive. Studies on cortisol have reported conflicting results, with a few showing an elevation of cortisol levels and others not, and intervention studies have been negative. A recent study showed that cortisol was increased in the evenings in some subjects who had OSA [104], consistent with findings in healthy subjects subjected to sleep restriction [32]. SDB may also influence the somatotropic axis, with some studies showing decreased levels of growth hormone [90] or IGF-1 [88,105] in OSA, which then increased after treatment with CPAP. The observations were dissimilar to the pattern of growth hormone secretion seen in experimental sleep restriction [32,33]. In relation to glucose tolerance, a decrease in growth hormone would be favorable, whereas a decrease in IGF-1 was reported to predict type 2 diabetes [106]. Given the complexity of growth hormone dynamics, the biologic significance of these observations in OSA in relation to glucose homeostasis remains speculative.

Hypoxia–reoxygenation in OSA may be a stimulus for insulin resistance and glucose intolerance. Using intermittent hypoxia exposure (30 seconds of hypoxia alternating with 30 seconds of normoxia for 16 hours in the 24-hour cycle) for 5 days and 12 weeks to simulate hypoxic stress of OSA, obese leptin-deficient mice developed a time-dependent worsening of insulin resistance and glucose intolerance that could be abolished by prior leptin infusion, whereas lean mice showed no change in insulin levels and an increase in leptin [107].

However, studies of circulating leptin levels in humans have conflicted, with some reporting increased leptin level in individuals who had OSA compared with those who did not [108,109], whereas others showed that the increase was only attributed to obesity rather than sleep apnea [110]. Another experimental model exposing HeLa cells to 5 minutes of hypoxia alternating with 10 minutes of normoxia showed up-regulation of the nuclear factor-κB pathway, which is involved in mediating inflammation and glucose transport and use [111]. Consistent with the up-regulation of this pathway, the study also reported an increase in plasma tumor necrosis factor (TNF) in individuals who had OSA. Although oxidative stress is considered a pathogenetic mechanism in diabetes mellitus [112], and increased oxidative stress has been repeatedly shown in subjects who have OSA [113–115], these findings are inconsistent [116]. Furthermore, the relationship of increased oxidative stress and glucose metabolism in OSA has not been explored.

Adipose tissue, and in particular visceral abdominal fat, is a rich source of adipokines and cytokines that influence insulin sensitivity. SDB may modulate the expression and secretion of these inflammatory mediators from fat and other tissue. Several studies have reported that individuals who had OSA had elevated levels of TNF-α or interleukin-6 [117,118], which are cytokines that are antagonistic to the actions of insulin [119,120]. Eventually more adipokines and adipocytokines will likely be explored for their role in glucose metabolism in OSA.

Summary

The sleep state itself has modulatory effects on glucose homeostasis. Epidemiologic and experimental studies suggest that sleep loss and sleep disturbances are detrimental to metabolic function and may predispose to obesity or glucose intolerance. Apart from the common risk factor of obesity, increasing data also support that OSA exerts independent adverse effects on glucose intolerance/diabetes mellitus, although definitive evidence is still needed.

Acknowledgments

The authors are grateful to Professor Eve Van Cauter of the University of Chicago for her support with the preparation of this manuscript.

References

[1] Gavin JR III, Alberti KGMM, Davidson MB, et al. Report of the expert committee on the diagnosis and classification of diabetes mellitus. Diabetes Care 1997;20:1183–97.

[2] American Diabetes Association. Diagnosis and classification of diabetes mellitus. Diabetes Care 2005;28(1):S37–42.

[3] Kahn CR, Saltiel AR. The molecular mechanism of insulin action and the regulation of glucose and lipid metabolism. In: Kahn CR, editor. Joslin's diabetes mellitus. 4th edition. Boston: Lippincott Williams & Wilkins; 2005. p. 145–68.

[4] Wilcox G. Insulin and insulin resistance. Clin Biochem Rev 2005;26(2):19–39.

[5] O'Rahilly S. Science, medicine, and the future. Non-insulin dependent diabetes mellitus: the gathering storm. BMJ 1997;314:955–9.

[6] World Health Organization. Diabetes mellitus: report of a WHO Study Group. Geneva (Switzerland): World Health Org; 1985 [Technical Report Series No. 727].

[7] Reaven GM. Insulin resistance, the insulin resistance syndrome, and cardiovascular disease. Panminerva Med 2005;47(4):201–10.

[8] Eckel R, Grundy S, Zimmet P. The metabolic syndrome. Lancet 2005;365(9468):1415–28.

[9] WHO Consultation Group. Definition, diagnosis and classification of diabetes mellitus and its complications. In: Alberti K, Zimmet P, editors. Part 1: diagnosis and classification of diabetes mellitus WHO/NCD/NCS/99. 2nd edition. Geneva (Switzerland): World Health Organization; 1999. p. 1–59.

[10] National Cholesterol Education Program. Third report of the expert panel on detection, evaluation, and treatment of high blood cholesterol in adults (adult treatment panel III) executive summary. 2001. Available at: http://www.nhlbi.nih.gov/guidelines/cholesterol/atp3full.pdf. Accessed December 2006.

[11] Goutham RAO. Insulin resistance syndrome. Am Fam Physician 2001;63(6):1159–63.

[12] Zimmet P, Alberti K. The changing face of marcovascular disease in non-insulin dependent diabetes mellitus in different cultures: an epidemic in progress. Lancet 1997;350:S1–4.

[13] Sicree R, Shaw JE, Zimmer PZ. The global burden of diabetes. In: Gan D, editor. Diabetes atlas. 2nd edition. Brussels (Belgium): International Diabetes Federation; 2003. p. 15–71.

[14] Zimmet P, Shaw J. Diabetes—a worldwide problem. In: Kahn RC, editor. Joslin's diabetes mellitus. 4th edition. Philadelphia: Lippincott Williams & Wilkins; 2005. p. 525–9.

[15] Van Cauter E, Polonsky KS, Scheen AJ. Roles of circadian rhythmicity and sleep in human glucose regulation. Endocr Rev 1997;18:716–38.

[16] Maquet P, Dive D, Salmon E, et al. Cerebral glucose utilization during stage 2 sleep in men. Brain Res 1992;571:149–53.

[17] Maquet P. Position omission tomography studies of sleep and sleep disorders. J Neurol 1997; 244:S23–8.

[18] Van Cauter E, Blackman JD, Roland D, et al. Modulation of glucose regulation and insulin secretion by circadian rhythmicity and sleep. J Clin Invest 1991;88:934–42.

[19] National Sleep Foundation. "Sleep in America" poll. Washington, DC: National Sleep Foundation; 2002.

[20] Jean-Louis G, Kripke DF, Ancoli-Israel S. Sleep and quality of well-being. Sleep 2000;23: 1115–21.

[21] National Center for Health Statistics. QuickStats: percentage of adults who reported an average of ≤ 6 hours of sleep per 24-hour period, by sex and age group–United States, 1985 and 2004. MMWR Morb Mortal Wkly Rep 2005;54(MM37):933.

[22] Ogden CL, Carroll MD, Curtin LR, et al. Prevalence of overweight and obesity in the United States, 1999-2004. JAMA 2006;295:1549–55.

[23] Ohayon MM. Epidemiology of insomnia: what we know and what we still need to learn. Sleep Med Rev 2002;6:97–111.

[24] Young T, Palta M, Dempsey J, et al. The occurrence of sleep-disordered breathing among middle-aged adults. N Engl J Med 1993; 328(17):1230–5.

[25] Rechtschaffen A, Gilliland MA, Bergmann BM, et al. Physiological correlates of prolonged sleep deprivation in rats. Science 1983; 221(4606):182–4.

[26] Rechtschaffen A, Bergmann BM, Everson CA, et al. Sleep deprivation in the rat: X. Integration and discussion of the findings. Sleep 1989;12: 68–87.

[27] VanHelder T, Symons JD, Radomski MW. Effects of sleep deprivation and exercise on glucose tolerance. Aviat Space Environ Med 1993; 64:487–92.

[28] Spiegel K, Leproult R, L'Hermite-Baleriaux M, et al. Leptin levels are dependent on sleep duration: relationships with sympathovagal balance, carbohydrate regulation, cortisol, and thyrotropin. J Clin Endocrinol Metab 2004;89: 5762–71.

[29] Kahn SE, Prigeon RL, McCulloch DK, et al. Quantification of the relationship between insulin sensitivity and beta-cell function in human subjects. Evidence for a hyperbolic function. Diabetes 1993;42:1663–72.

[30] Catalano PM, Tyzbir ED, Wolfe RR, et al. Carbohydrate metabolism during pregnancy in control subjects and women with gestational diabetes. Am J Physiol 1993;264:E60–7.

[31] Spiegel K, Tasali E, Penev P, et al. Brief communication: sleep curtailment in healthy young men is associated with decreased leptin levels, elevated ghrelin levels, and increased hunger and appetite. Ann Intern Med 2004;141(11): 846–50.

[32] Spiegel K, Leproult R, Van Cauter E. Impact of sleep debt on metabolic and endocrine function. Lancet 1999;354:1435–9.

[33] Spiegel K, Leproult R, Colecchia EF, et al. Adaptation of the 24-h growth hormone profile to

a state of sleep debt. Am J Physiol Regul Integr Comp Physiol 2000;279:R874–83.

[34] Irwin MR, Wang M, Campomayor CO, et al. Sleep deprivation and activation of morning levels of cellular and genomic markers of inflammation. Arch Intern Med 2006;166:1756–62.

[35] Festa A, D'Agostino R Jr, Howard G, et al. Chronic subclinical inflammation as part of the insulin resistance syndrome: the Insulin Resistance Atherosclerosis Study (IRAS). Circulation 2000;102:42–7.

[36] Vgontzas AN, Zoumakis E, Bixler EO, et al. Adverse effects of modest sleep restriction on sleepiness, performance, and inflammatory cytokines. J Clin Endocrinol Metab 2004;89:2119–26.

[37] Knutson K, Spiegel K, Penev P, et al. Metabolic consequences of sleep deprivation. Sleep Med Rev, in press.

[38] Gottlieb DJ, Punjabi NM, Newman AB, et al. Association of sleep time with diabetes mellitus and impaired glucose tolerance. Arch Intern Med 2005;165:863–8.

[39] Ayas NT, White DP, Al-Delaimy WK, et al. A prospective study of self-reported sleep duration and incident diabetes in women. Diabetes Care 2003;26:380–4.

[40] Yaggi HK, Araujo AB, McKinlay JB. Sleep duration as a risk factor for the development of type 2 diabetes. Diabetes Care 2006;29(3):657–61.

[41] Mallon L, Browman JE, Hetta J. High incidence of diabetes in men with sleep complaints or short sleep duration; a 12-year follow-up study of a middle-aged population. Diabetes Care 2005;28:2762–7.

[42] Bjorkelund C, Bondyr-Carlsson D, Lapidus L, et al. Sleep disturbances in midlife unrelated to 32-year diabetes incidence: the prospective population study of women in Gothenburg. Diabetes Care 2005;28:2739–44.

[43] Nilsson PM, Roost M, Engstrom G, et al. Incidence of diabetes in middle-aged men is related to sleep disturbances. Diabetes Care 2004; 27(10):2464–9.

[44] Kawakami N, Takatsuka N, Shimizu H. Sleep disturbance and onset of type 2 diabetes. Diabetes Care 2004;27:282–3.

[45] Meisinger C, Heier M, Loewel H, et al. Sleep disturbance as a predictor of type 2 diabetes mellitus in men and women from the general population. Diabetologia 2005;48:235–41.

[46] Gislason T, Almiqvist M. Somatic diseases and sleep complaints: an epidemiologic study of 3201 Swedish men. Acta Med Scand 1987;221: 475–81.

[47] Hyyppa MT, Khronholm E. Quality of sleep and chronic illnesses. J Clin Epidemiol 1989;42:633–8.

[48] Sridhar GR, Madhu K. Prevalence of sleep disturbances in diabetes mellitus. Diabetes Res Clin Pract 1994;23:183–6.

[49] Lamond N, Tiggemann M, Dawson D. Facotrs predicting sleep disruption type II diabetes. Sleep 2000;23:415–6.

[50] Knutson KL, Ryden AM, Mander BA, et al. Role of sleep duration and quality in the risk and severity of type II diabetes mellitus. Arch Intern Med 2006;166:1768–74.

[51] Shigeta H, Shigeta M, Nakazawa A, et al. Lifestyle. Obesity and insulin resistance. Diabetes Care 2001;24(3):608.

[52] Sekine M, Yamagami T, Handa K, et al. A dose-response relationship between short sleeping hours and childhood obesity: results of the Toyama Birth Cohort Study. Child Care Health Dev 2002;28:163–70.

[53] Vorona RD, Winn MP, Babineau TW, et al. Overweight and obese patients in a primary care population report less sleep than patients with a normal body mass index. Arch Intern Med 2005;165:25–30.

[54] Taheri S, Lin L, Austin D, et al. Short sleep duration is associated with reduced leptin, elevated ghrelin, and increased body mass index. PLoS Med 2004;1(3):211–7.

[55] Young T, Peppard P, Gottlieb D. Epidemiology of obstructive sleep apnea. A population health perspective. Am J Respir Crit Care Med 2002; 165:1217–39.

[56] Lam B, Lam DCL, Ip MSM. Obstructive sleep apnea in Asia. Int J Tuberc Lung Dis 2007; 11(1):2–11.

[57] Hiestand DM, Britz P, Goldman M, et al. Prevalence of symptoms and risk of sleep apnea in the US population: results from the National Sleep Foundation Sleep in America 2005 poll. Chest 2006;130(3):780–6.

[58] Jennum P, Schultz-Larsen K, Christensen N. Snoring sympathetic activity and cardiovascular risk factors in a 70 year old population. Eur J Epidemiol 1993;9:477–82.

[59] Grunstein RR, Stenlof K, Hedner J, et al. Impact of obstructive sleep apnea and sleepiness on metabolic and cardiovascular risk factors in the Swedish obese subjects (SOS) study. Int J Obes Relat Metab Disord 1995;19:410–8.

[60] Enright PL, Newman AB, Wahl PW, et al. Prevalence and correlates of snoring and observed apneas in 5201 older adults. Sleep 1996;19: 531–8.

[61] Renko AK, Hiltunen L, Laakso M, et al. The relationship of glucose tolerance to sleep disorders and daytime sleepiness. Diabetes Res Clin Pract 2005;67:84–91.

[62] Shin C, Kim J, Kim J, et al. Association of habitual snoring with glucose and insulin metabolism in nonobese Korean adult men. Am J Respir Crit Care Med 2005;171(3):287–91.

[63] Elmasry A, Lindberg E, Berne C, et al. Sleep-disordered breathing and glucose metabolism in hypertensive men, a population-based study. J Intern Med 2001;249:153–61.

[64] Punjabi NM, Sorkin JD, Katzel LI, et al. Sleep-disordered breathing and insulin resistance in middle-aged and overweight men. Am J Respir Crit Care Med 2002;165:677–82.

[65] Punjabi NM, Shahar E, Redline S, et al. Sleep-disordered breathing, glucose intolerance, and insulin resistance: the Sleep Heart Health Study. Am J Epidemiol 2004;160(6):521–30.

[66] Resnick HE, Redline S, Shahar E, et al. Diabetes and sleep disturbances. Diabetes Care 2003;26: 702–9.

[67] Punjabi NM, Ahmed MM, Polotsky VY, et al. Sleep-disordered breathing, glucose intolerance, and insulin resistance. Respir Physiol Neurobiol 2003;136:167–78.

[68] Punjabi NM, Polotsky VY. Disorders of glucose metabolism in sleep apnea. J Appl Physiol 2005;99:1998–2007.

[69] Tiihonen M, Partinen M, Narvanen S. The severity of obstructive sleep apnoea is associated with insuin resistance. J Sleep Res 1993;2: 56–61.

[70] Vgontzas AN, Papanicolaou DA, Bixler EO, et al. Sleep apnea and daytime sleepiness and fatigue: relation to visceral obesity, insulin resistance, and hypercytokinemia. J Clin Endocrinol Metab 2000;85:1151–8.

[71] Davies RJO, Turner R, Crosby J, et al. Plasma insulin and lipid levels in untreated obstructive sleep apnoea and snoring; their comparison with matched controls and response to treatment. J Sleep Res 1994;3:180–5.

[72] Stoohs RA, Facchini F, Guilleminault C. Insulin resistance and sleep-disordered breathing in healthy humans. Am J Respir Crit Care Med 1996;154:170–4.

[73] Strohl KP, Novak RD, Singer W, et al. Insulin levels, blood pressure and sleep apnea. Sleep 1994;17:614–8.

[74] Ip MSM, Lam B, Ng MMT, et al. Obstructive sleep apnea is independently associated with insulin resistance. Am J Respir Crit Care Med 2002;165:670–6.

[75] Tassone F, Lanfranco F, Gianotti L, et al. Obstructive sleep apnoea syndrome impairs insulin sensitivity independently of anthropometric variables. Clin Endocrinol 2003;59:374–9.

[76] Sasanabe R, Katsuhisa B, Otake K, et al. Metabolic syndrome in Japanese patients with obstructive sleep apnea syndrome. Hypertens Res 2006;29:315–22.

[77] Coughlin SR, Mawdsley L, Mugarza JA, et al. Obstructive sleep apnea is independently associated with an increased prevalence of metabolic syndrome. Eur Heart J 2004;25:735–41.

[78] West SD, Nicoll DJ, Stradling JR. Prevalence of obstructive sleep apnoea in men with type 2 diabetes. Thorax 2006;61(11):945–50.

[79] de la Eva RC, Baur LA, Donaghue KC, et al. Metabolic correlates with obstructive sleep apnea in obese subjects. J Pediatr 2002;140:654–9.

[80] Tauman R, O'Brien LM, Ivanenko A, et al. Obesity rather than severity of sleep-disordered breathing as the major determinant of insulin resistance and altered lipidemia in snoring children. Pediatrics 2005;116(1):e66–73.

[81] Kaditis AG, Alexopoulos EI, Damani E, et al. Obstructive sleep-disordered breathing and fasting insulin levels in nonobese children. Pediatr Pulmonol 2005;40(6):515–23.

[82] Elmasry A, Janson C, Lindberg E, et al. The role of habitual snoring and obesity in the development of diabetes, a 10-year follow-up study in a male population. J Intern Med 2000;248:13–20.

[83] Al-Delaimy WK, Manson JE, Willett WC, et al. Snoring as a risk factor for type II diabetes mellitus: a prospective study. Am J Epidemiol 2002; 55:387–93.

[84] Reichmuth KJ, Austin D, Skatrud JB, et al. Association of sleep apnea and type II diabetes: a population-based study. Am J Respir Crit Care Med 2005;172(12):1590–5.

[85] Brooks B, Cistulli PA, Borkman M, et al. Obstructive sleep apnea in obese noninsulin-dependent diabetic patients: effect of continuous positive airway pressure treatment on insulin responsiveness. J Clin Endocrinol Metab 1994; 79:1681–5.

[86] Chin K, Nakamuta T, Takahashi K, et al. Effects of obstructive sleep apnea syndrome on serum amiotransfease levels in obese patients. Am J Med 2003;114(5):370–6.

[87] Chin K, Shimizu K, Nakamura T, et al. Changes in intra-abdominal visceral fat and serum leptin levels in patients with obstructive sleep apnea syndrome following nasal continuous positive airway pressure therapy. Circulation 1999;100: 706–12.

[88] Cooper BG, White JE, Ashworth LA, et al. Hormonal and metabolic profiles in subjects with obstructive sleep apnea syndrome and the acute effects of nasal continuous positive airway pressure (CPAP) treatment. Sleep 1995;18:172–9.

[89] Saarelainen S, Lahtela J, Kallonen E. Effect of nasal CPAP treatment on insulin sensitivity and plasma leptin. J Sleep Res 1997;6:146–7.

[90] Saini J, Krieger J, Brandenberger G, et al. Continuous positive airway pressure treatment. Effects on growth hormone, insulin and glucose profiles in obstructive sleep apnea patients. Horm Metab Res 1993;25:375–81.

[91] Smurra M, Philip P, Thaillard J, et al. CPAP treatment does not affect glucose-insulin metabolism in sleep apneic patients. Sleep Med 2001;2:207–13.

[92] Stoohs RA, Facchini FS, Phillp P, et al. Selected cardiovascular risk factors in patients with obstructive sleep apnea: effect of nasal continuous positive airway pressure (n-CPAP). Sleep 1993; 16:S141–2.

[93] Harsch IA, Schahin SP, Radespiel-Troger M, et al. Continuous positive airway pressure treatment rapidly improves insulin sensitivity in patients with obstructive sleep apnea syndrome. Am J Respir Crit Care Med 2004;169:156–62.

[94] Babu AR, Herdegen J, Fogelfeld L, et al. Type 2 diabetes, glycemic control, and continuous

positive airway pressure in obstructive sleep apnea. Arch Intern Med 2005;165(4):447–52.

[95] Hassaballa HA, Tulaimat A, Herdegen JJ, et al. The effect of continuous positive airway pressure on glucose control in diabetic patients with severe obstructive sleep apnea. Sleep Breath 2005;9:176–80.

[96] Lindberg E, Berne C, Elmasry A, et al. CPAP treatment of a population-based sample—what are the benefits and the treatment compliance? Sleep Med 2006;7:553–60.

[97] West SD, Nicoll DJ, Wallace TM, et al. Obstructive sleep apnoea in men with type 2 diabetes: a double blind randomized controlled trial of the effects of CPAP on HbA1c and insulin resistance. Proc Amer Thor Soc 2006;3:A733.

[98] Spiegel K, Knutson K, Leproult R, et al. Sleep loss: a novel risk factor for insulin resistance and Type 2 diabetes. J Appl Physiol 2005;99: 2008–19.

[99] Somers VK, Narkiewicz K. Sympathetic nerve activity in obstructive sleep apnoea. Acta Physiol Scand 2003;177(3):385–90.

[100] Dimsdale JE, Coy T, Ziegler MG, et al. The effect of sleep apnea on plasma and urinary catecholamines. Sleep 1995;18(5):377–81.

[101] Marrone O, Riccobono L, Salvaggio A, et al. Catecholamines and blood pressure in obstructive sleep apnea syndrome. Chest 1993;103:722–7.

[102] Leuenberger U, Jacob E, Sweer L, et al. Surges of muscle sympathetic nerve activity during obstructive apnea are linked to hypoxemia. J Appl Physiol 1995;79(2):581–8.

[103] Lam JCM, Tam S, Ooi CG, et al. Relationship between sympathetic activity, obesity, and obstructive sleep apnea. Sleep Med 2006; 7(Suppl 2):S51.

[104] Parlapiano C, Borgia MC, Minni A, et al. Cortisol circadian rhythm and 24-hour Holter arterial pressure in OSAS patients. Endocr Res 2005; 31(4):371–4.

[105] Grunstein RR, Handelsman DJ, Lawrence SJ, et al. Neuroendocrine dysfunction in sleep apnea: reversal by continuous positive airways pressure therapy. J Clin Endocrinol Metab 1989; 68(2):352–8.

[106] Sandhu MS, Heald AH, Gibson JM, et al. Circulating concentrations of insulin-like growth factor-I and development of glucose intolerance: a prospective observational study. Lancet 2002; 359:1740–5.

[107] Polotsky VY, Li J, Punjabi NM, et al. Intermittent hypoxia increases insulin resistance in genetically obese mice. J Physiol 2003;552(1): 253–64.

[108] Philips BG, Kato M, Narkiewicz K, et al. Increases in leptin levels, sympathetic drive, and weight gain in obstructive sleep apnea. Am J Physiol Heart Circ Physiol 2000;279(1):H234–7.

[109] Ip MSM, Lam KSL, Ho CM, et al. Serum leptin and vascular risk factors in obstructive sleep apnea. Chest 2000;118:580–6.

[110] Schafer H, Pauleit D, Sudhop T, et al. Body fat distribution, serum leptin, and cardiovascular risk factors in men with obstructive sleep apnea. Chest 2002;122:829–39.

[111] Ryan S, Taylor CT, McNicholas WT. Selective activation of inflammatory pathways by intermittent hypoxia in obstructive sleep apnea syndrome. Circulation 2005;112(17):2660–7.

[112] Nourooz-Zadeh J, Rahimi A, Tajaddini-Sarmadi J, et al. Relationships between plasma measures of oxidative stress and metabolic control in NIDDM. Diabetologia 1997;40:647–53.

[113] Lavie L. Obstructive sleep apnea syndrome—an oxidative stress disorder. Sleep Med Rev 2003; 7(1):33–51.

[114] Dyugovskaya L, Lavie P, Lavie L. Increased adhesion molecules expression and production of reactive oxygen species in leukocytes of sleep apnea patients. Am J Respir Crit Care Med 2002; 165:934–9.

[115] Schulz R, Mahmoudi S, Hattar K, et al. Enhanced release of superoxide from polymophonuclear neutrophils in obstructive sleep apnea. Impact of continuous positive airway pressure therapy. Am J Respir Crit Care Med 2000;162: 566–70.

[116] Svatikova A, Wolk R, Lerman LO, et al. Oxidative stress in obstructive sleep apnea. Eur Heart J 2005;26(22):2435–9.

[117] Vgontzas AN, Legro RS, Bixler EO, et al. Elevation of plasma cytokines in disorders of excessive daytime sleepiness: role of sleep disturbance and obesity. J Clin Endocrinol Metab 1997;2(5): 1313–6.

[118] Vgontzas AN, Bixler EO, Chrousos GP. Metabolic disturbances in obesity versus sleep apnea: the importance of visceral obesity and insulin resistance. J Intern Med 2003;254(1): 32–44.

[119] Hotamisligil GS, Shargill NS, Spiegelman BM. Adipose expression of tumor necrosis factor-α: direct role in obesity-linked insulin resistance. Science 1993;259:87–91.

[120] Bastard JP, Maachi M, Tran Van Nheiu J, et al. Adipose tissue IL-6 content correlates with resistance to insulin activation of glucose uptake both in vivo and in vitro. J Clin Endocrinol metab 2002;87:2084–9.

ELSEVIER
SAUNDERS

SLEEP
MEDICINE
CLINICS

Sleep Med Clin 2 (2007) 31–39

Sleep Disturbance in Fibromyalgia

Margaret D. Lineberger, PhD[a],*, Melanie K. Means, PhD[a,b],
Jack D. Edinger, PhD[a,b]

- Nature and significance of sleep
  disturbance in fibromyalgia
  Subjective sleep complaints
  Objective sleep findings
  *Alpha electroencephalogram sleep
  anomaly*
- Pathophysiology of sleep disturbance
  in fibromyalgia
- Management of sleep difficulties
  in fibromyalgia
  Pharmacologic treatments
  Nonpharmacologic treatments
  Multidisciplinary treatment
- Summary
- References

Fibromyalgia (FM), characterized by diffuse myalgia, multiple topographically specific tender points, chronic fatigue, psychosocial distress, and disturbed, unrefreshing sleep, is a prevalent and significant health problem. Surveys suggest that between 0.5% and 10.5% of the general population suffer from this disorder, and 5% to 6% of all patients seen in general and family medicine clinics present FM complaints to their physicians [1–11]. Moreover, FM is the third most common disorder encountered in specialty rheumatology clinics, and accounts for roughly 15% of all patients seen in such settings [11,12]. Although the FM diagnosis remains controversial among practitioners, both clinical and epidemiological findings suggest considerable morbidity may be associated with this condition. At a minimum, FM results in chronic discomfort/pain, daytime fatigue, decreased mood, and general malaise [13]. In more protracted cases this condition may lead to increased absenteeism from work, reduced vocational and domestic functioning, enhanced health care costs, and in extreme cases, chronic disability [14–19]. Thus

patients presenting FM complaints warrant early, effective treatment.

Of all FM symptoms, sleep disturbance is among the more common, and perhaps more etiologically significant. Indeed, clinical survey studies suggest that the majority of all FM patients present with insomnia complaints, including difficulty initiating sleep, sleep maintenance problems, or persistent nonrestorative sleep [20–25]. Corroborating these subjective complaints are numerous objective, polysomnographic studies that have shown excessive wake time, increased arousals, and the intrusion of waking-like alpha electroencephalogram (EEG) frequencies into nonrapid eye movement (NREM) sleep (ie, the alpha-delta sleep pattern) to be common among FM patients [26–30]. Moreover, various studies suggest that this sleep pathology may play a substantial role in perpetuating not only the general fatigue and malaise of FM patients, but also their generalized physical discomfort and pain. Studies of clinical FM patients have shown that a worsening of sleep enhances subsequent daytime distress and pain complaints, whereas

[a] Department of Psychiatry and Behavioral Sciences, Duke University Medical Center, Box 2908, Durham, NC 27710, USA
[b] Veterans Affairs Medical Center (116B), 508 Fulton Street, Durham, NC 27705, USA
* Corresponding author.
E-mail address: meg.lineberger@duke.edu (M.D. Lineberger).

doi:10.1016/j.jsmc.2006.11.006

exacerbations of daytime pain or psychosocial distress often are followed by increased nocturnal sleep disruption [31–36]. Given such findings, it seems reasonable to speculate that sleep disturbance is mechanistically important to the etiology or symptom maintenance of the FM syndrome. This article provides an overview of FM-related sleep difficulties and their treatment.

Nature and significance of sleep disturbance in fibromyalgia

Subjective sleep complaints

It is widely recognized that sleep disturbance is a highly common and significant component of the FM syndrome. In fact, the American College of Rheumatology criteria for the classification of fibromyalgia identify sleep disturbance as a central associated symptom of FM, occurring in 73% to 76% of FM patients in a clinical sample; only fatigue and morning stiffness were reported more frequently [17]. Hence, the nature, significance, and management of sleep difficulties among FM sufferers have been a primary concern for clinicians and researchers alike.

To date, both anecdotal clinical observations and systematic studies of FM patients have shown that FM patients present varied and significant sleep complaints. Clinical observations show that FM patients commonly complain of insomnia symptoms such as difficulties initiating or maintaining sleep. Formal studies employing the Pittsburgh Sleep Quality Index (PSQI), a well-validated psychometric instrument for assessing sleep disturbance, have shown that FM patients score well above the clinical cutoff that connotes general sleep pathology. PSQI subscore analyses also have shown that FM patients report longer sleep latencies, more sleep fragmentation, and greater associated daytime dysfunction than do matched normal sleepers [37]. Moreover, the total PSQI score is significantly negatively correlated with pain threshold in FM patients [38]. Thus, the insomnia symptoms of FM patients appear significant both considered in isolation and in the context of the larger FM syndrome.

Along with classic insomnia symptoms, FM patients commonly complain of persistent, nonrestorative sleep, or sleep that is perceived as light, unrefreshing, or of poor quality despite what may be a normal duration. This is perhaps the most common FM-associated sleep complaint, in that up to 100% of all FM patients report at least intermittent problems with nonrestorative sleep [23]. Studies conducted in the general population suggest that subjective complaints of nonrestorative sleep are associated with greater daytime impairment (eg, fatigue, irritable mood) compared with other insomnia complaints [39]. In FM, nonrestorative sleep may contribute to other FM symptoms, including increased pain, pain awareness, and daytime fatigue. When prospective daily ratings of pain and sleep quality have been collected from FM patients, within-person changes in sleep quality have been found to predict changes in pain from day to day [32], whereas poor sleep quality mediated the relationship between pain and fatigue [21]. As such, this form of sleep difficulty may play a mechanistic role in the cardinal daytime FM symptoms.

Objective sleep findings

Objective measurement of sleep in FM patients supports the subjective experience of nocturnal sleep disturbance. Motor activity monitoring of FM patients with actigraphy shows significantly increased activity levels at night compared with controls [40], and polysomnography in FM patients confirms significant alterations in sleep architecture, including increased stage 1 sleep, decreased slow wave sleep, and an overall increase in number of arousals [24,41]. The severity of these polysomnographic alternations are significantly correlated with daytime hypersomnolence, as documented by the Epworth Sleepiness Scale [42].

Alpha electroencephalogram sleep anomaly

Hauri and Hawkins [43] first described "alpha-delta sleep" as the intrusion of alpha waves (normally associated with relaxed wakefulness) superimposed on the delta frequency of slow wave sleep. Initially observed among patients who have chronic somatic complaints and fatigue [43], the alpha EEG sleep anomaly has been noted throughout NREM sleep in FM patients, and is associated with the subjective experience of shallow or nonrefreshing sleep [25–27,29,33,44]. Moreover, stage 4 sleep deprivation among healthy controls induces musculoskeletal and mood symptoms similar to those observed in FM patients [27]. These findings invited speculation that abnormal alpha activity in FM patients may interfere with the restorative function of NREM sleep, leading to increased daytime symptoms. The possibility of a biological marker for FM generated a great deal of interest in the relationship between sleep and pain in FM and related syndromes. Others, however, have reported that the alpha EEG sleep anomaly is neither sensitive nor specific to chronic pain conditions, because it also occurs in patients who have nonpainful medical or psychiatric illness [45,46]. In a recent study of more than 1000 sleep patients, only 5% exhibited alpha-delta sleep on polysomnography, and fewer than 40% of those reported chronic pain [46].

Pathophysiology of sleep disturbance in fibromyalgia

The specific etiology of FM is unknown, but research implicates heightened central nervous system (CNS) sensitization and endocrine abnormalities, leading to increased pain sensitivity [47]. Despite the relative prevalence of nonrestorative sleep among FM patients, abnormal sleep architecture is unlikely to be a direct pathophysiologic mechanism for FM. As noted above, the alpha EEG sleep anomaly lacks sensitivity and specificity as a biological marker for FM. Sleep does play a role in a multifactorial model of FM, however. When prospective ratings are made of pain, sleep quality, and fatigue, two alternate models have emerged: (1) increased pain interferes with sleep quality, resulting in increased fatigue the next day [21]; and (2) poor sleep quality leads to increased pain *and* fatigue the next day [32]. Taken together, these models point to a disruptive cycle in which pain and sleep interact reciprocally to influence symptom presence and severity.

Management of sleep difficulties in fibromyalgia

Because there is no single treatment for FM, management of this disorder often requires an integrative symptom-focused approach incorporating both pharmacologic and nonpharmacologic therapies. In addition to effective analgesic relief, treatments targeting sleep difficulties often prove beneficial. As noted above, pain and sleep disturbance in FM may interact in a reciprocal manner—pain disrupts sleep and exacerbates sleep problems that, in turn, perpetuate daytime symptoms such as fatigue and pain [32,48]. In addition, careful assessment of the sleep complaint is warranted to evaluate for the presence of a comorbid primary sleep disorder, because FM may be associated with sleep-disordered breathing or sleep-related movement disorders such as restless legs syndrome or periodic limb movement disorder [24,47,49–51]. Although there are no specific treatments for sleep difficulties in FM, pharmacologic and nonpharmacologic interventions can provide symptomatic benefit.

Pharmacologic treatments

A variety of pharmacologic agents are available for treating sleep disturbance in FM. Sedative-hypnotic medications are commonly used to treat insomnia and may improve the sleep of FM patients. Antidepressant medications and muscle relaxants may target other symptoms such as mood or pain but have secondary effects on sleep. A number of additional pharmacologic agents also have shown beneficial effects on the sleep patterns of FM patients. Each of these pharmacologic approaches is considered in some detail in the following discussion.

Sedative hypnotics

Benzodiazepines such as temazepam can ameliorate the sleep disturbance of FM patients [52]; however, the newer nonbenzodiazepine hypnotics have become a popular treatment for insomnia because of their improved side-effect profile compared with traditional benzodiazepines. In FM patients, both zoplicone and zolpidem improve subjective ratings of sleep disturbance and daytime energy compared with placebo, but do not impact pain levels [53–55]. Despite subjective sleep improvements reported by FM patients, zoplicone does not alter the sleep architecture measured via polysomnography [53].

Sodium oxybate is a formulation of gamma-hydroxybutyrate (GHB), an endogenous CNS metabolite. It is a CNS depressant, approved by the Food and Drug Administration (FDA) for the treatment of narcolepsy with cataplexy. GHB has been found to stimulate slow wave sleep and growth hormone secretion in healthy individuals [56]. Because FM patients exhibit both decreased slow wave sleep and low growth hormone secretion, the effect of sodium oxybate on the sleep patterns of FM patients has been investigated [57]. Compared with placebo, FM patients taking sodium oxybate demonstrated objective polysomnographic sleep improvements such as increased slow wave sleep, decreased sleep latency, and reduced alpha EEG sleep anomaly, along with a self-reported enhancement in sleep quality. Sodium oxybate also was associated with improvements in pain and fatigue symptoms. It is important to note, however, that this medication has not been approved for use in patients who have FM.

Melatonin, a hormone synthesized by the pineal gland, influences the organization of circadian rhythms. Interest in the relationship between endogenous melatonin secretion and FM has yielded inconsistent findings [58–60]. Although not FDA-approved, melatonin is widely available as a nutritional supplement and has become a popular over-the-counter remedy for insomnia. Case reports [61] and one open-label pilot study [62] with FM patients suggest some sleep improvements subsequent to melatonin therapy; however, the lack of controlled trials, along with a failure to detect circadian abnormalities in individuals who have FM, do not support the use of melatonin as a sleep aid in FM [63,64].

Antidepressant medications

Antidepressants are commonly used to treat FM, and include tricyclic antidepressants (TCAs), selective serotonin reuptake inhibitors (SSRIs), dual reuptake inhibitors, and monoamine oxidase inhibitors [65]. Two meta-analyses have shown that such antidepressants produce a moderate effect on sleep in FM patients [66,67]. The combination of an SSRI such as fluoxetine with a TCA such as amitriptyline may confer benefits to sleep beyond either medication alone [68]. The alpha EEG sleep anomaly does not seem to predict response to antidepressant treatment [66,69]; however, preliminary findings suggest that the atypical antidepressant trazodone increases slow wave sleep and reduces the alpha EEG sleep anomaly in FM patients [70].

Muscle relaxants

Muscle relaxants prescribed for pain or muscle tension, such as cyclobenzaprine, carisoprodol, and tizanidine, may have sedating effects as well [65,71]. Cyclobenzaprine is commonly used to treat FM and has a pharmacologic structure similar to TCAs. It appears to have few specific effects on sleep physiology and does not alter the alpha EEG sleep anomaly in FM patients [72]. Nonetheless, a number of studies have found that subjective sleep disturbance, at least in the short-term, improves subsequent to cyclobenzaprine [73–76]. Furthermore, sleep may respond favorably to low doses, reducing the likelihood of side effects [65]. A recent meta-analysis of its effects on FM symptoms suggested that cyclobenzaprine was associated with moderate improvements in sleep over 12 weeks, although individuals in the placebo conditions also experienced similar sleep improvements [77].

Other medications

Pregabalin is an anti-epileptic medication that is FDA-approved for the management of neuropathic pain conditions. It may confer particular benefit to FM patients, because it has been found to enhance slow wave sleep while reducing sleep-onset latency and number of awakenings in healthy volunteers [78]. In a randomized controlled study with FM patients [79], pregabalin was associated with self-reported reductions in sleep problems and improvement in sleep quality compared with placebo.

Tropisetron, a highly-selective serotonin receptor antagonist, is typically prescribed as an antiemetic. Although not available in the United States, European researchers have reported sleep-related benefits in FM patients treated with tropisetron [80–84]. Other pharmacologic agents such as quetiapine (an atypical antipsychotic) [85] and sibutramine hydrochloride monohydrate (marketed for the treatment of obesity) [86] have been linked to sleep improvements in some individuals who have FM, but controlled studies have not been conducted.

Nonpharmacologic treatments

Pharmacologic treatments may be inadequate in resolving sleep difficulties in FM. Patients may be particularly sensitive to the side effects of medications, or the benefits of such medications may not endure over time to provide sustained relief. Fortunately, nonpharmacologic strategies addressing sleep problems in FM are evolving and hold promise for improving sleep in FM patients.

Cognitive behavioral therapies

Cognitive behavioral therapies (CBT) for FM typically combines elements of education, skills training, and skills application to influence the thoughts and behaviors related to the experience of pain [87]. Although such therapies are beneficial in treating FM, they may not influence sleep patterns [88]. In the past decade, a cognitive behavioral therapy specific to insomnia (CBTI) has emerged as a frontline treatment for insomnia, and has shown application to a wide range of insomnias secondary to medical or psychiatric disorders [89]. CBTI involves a specific set of strategies designed to target psychological and behavioral factors that perpetuate sleep disturbance [90]. In a recent randomized controlled trial with FM, patients treated with CBTI experienced significant sleep improvements in both subjective and objective measures [91].

Exercise

Exercise is one of the most common nonpharmacologic treatments in FM, and is generally studied in relation to its benefit in reducing FM-related pain [92,93]. Although exercise typically enhances sleep in good sleepers, few studies of exercise in FM patients have considered sleep outcomes. The results of such investigations are inconsistent, but suggest that exercise may have some benefits to the sleep of FM patients [87,93–95].

Dietary modifications/supplements

Despite the popularity of dietary modifications among FM patients, such interventions have not been well-studied [96]. Not surprisingly, therefore, little is known about the effect of diet on sleep in FM. Some evidence suggests that subjective sleep improvements are associated with antioxidant food supplements or the adoption of a cholesterol-free vegan diet [97,98]. Dietary supplements containing tryptophan compounds have received some attention, given that tryptophan is a serotonin precursor that enhances sleepiness. In FM patients,

L-tryptophan does not alter slow wave sleep, alpha EEG sleep, pain, or mood symptoms [33]. Preliminary evidence suggests that a similar compound, 5-Hydroxytryptophan, may improve sleep quality in FM patients [99,100]; however, safety concerns surrounding tryptophan supplements have been present following a 1989 outbreak of eosinophilic myalgia syndrome in the United States resulting from a contaminated product.

Complementary and alternative therapies

Complementary and alternative therapies are often sought by individuals who have FM, perhaps reflecting the inadequacy of mainstream medical treatment [101]. Most of these therapies have not been rigorously evaluated in FM patients. Sleep improvements have been linked to hypnosis [102], yoga [103], chiropractic manipulations [104,105], acupuncture [105], homeopathic remedies [106], and therapeutic baths [94,105].

A variety of electrotherapies have been tested in FM patients. Among these, subjective sleep improvements have been reported with electro-acupuncture [107], EEG-driven stimulation (EEG biofeedback with photic stimulation) [108], low power laser [109], and a combination of ultrasound and interferential current [110]. In the latter study, treatment was associated with a number of sleep improvements on polysomnography, including reduced sleep fragmentation and increased slow wave sleep [110].

Multidisciplinary treatment

Multidisciplinary treatments typically combine elements of patient education, cognitive behavioral therapy, exercise, and pharmacotherapy; some experts also advocate the addition of a sleep hygiene component [71,111]. Initial evidence suggests that sleep may respond favorably to such approaches. In one study, a 10-week FM treatment program consisting of pool exercise and psychoeducation (including sleep hygiene and group biofeedback) was associated with greater sleep improvements compared with a control group and an exercise-only group [112]. Similarly, a pilot study of an 8-week program combining education, relaxation/mindfulness meditation, and qigong movement therapy was associated with self-reported sleep improvements [113]. Another study treating FM patients with amitriptyline combined with either a support group or a CBT pain group reported greater sleep improvements in the CBT group [114].

Summary

FM is a syndrome characterized by diffuse pain, fatigue, sleep complaints, and psychosocial distress. It is a prevalent and significant health problem, conferring considerable morbidity upon its patients. FM patients report clinically significant sleep disturbance, namely persistent, nonrestorative sleep. Polysomnography confirms significant alterations in sleep architecture in FM, and spectral analysis has shown intrusion of alpha waves throughout sleep, although this finding is neither sensitive nor specific to FM patients. Sleep disturbance may have etiological significance for FM, in that pain and sleep interact reciprocally to influence other cardinal symptoms of FM, including fatigue and psychological distress. There is currently no consensus for managing sleep disturbance in FM; however, symptom-focused interventions include both pharmacologic and nonpharmacologic therapies. Sedative hypnotics and antidepressant medications are commonly used to treat insomnia and associated FM symptoms, and there is increasing evidence for using cognitive behavioral interventions to improve sleep in FM patients.

In the 3 decades since Moldofsky and colleagues [27] first reported the alpha-EEG sleep anomaly among FM patients, research on the subjective and objective characteristics of sleep disturbance in FM has flourished; however, inconsistencies abound, with respect to both the definition of FM and the measurement of sleep variables. Future research in this area would benefit from more widespread adoption of research diagnostic criteria for FM [17] and insomnia [115], and the use of standardized measures of fatigue, sleep quality, and sleep parameters.

Similarly, given the prevalence of sleep complaints among this patient group, more information is needed on how to best manage the sleep problems among patients who have FM, and whether treatment designed to correct sleep disturbance in FM may interrupt the vicious sleep-pain/distress feedback cycle, and lead to overall symptom improvement. Pharmacologic studies show that many FM treatment gains tend to diminish substantially over time, with many patients returning to baseline levels of sleep difficulty, pain, and general dysfunction by scheduled follow-ups. These studies imply that symptom-oriented, pharmacologic approaches may produce only limited or transitory FM improvements, because they do not adequately address those mechanisms that perpetuate the long-term sleep difficulties of FM patients. More research is needed on whether nonpharmacologic treatments such as CBTI are superior to usual medical care for the management of multiple FM symptoms. Specifically, sleep improvements realized via CBTI could translate into lasting reductions in pain or mood disturbance/distress among FM sufferers.

References

[1] Wolfe F, Ross K, Anderson J, et al. The prevalence and characteristics of fibromyalgia in the general population. Arthritis Rheum 1995;38(1):19–28.

[2] Wallace DJ. Systemic lupus erythematosus, rheumatology and medical literature: current trends. J Rheumatol 1985;12(5):913–5.

[3] White KP, Thompson J. Fibromyalgia syndrome in an Amish community: a controlled study to determine disease and symptom prevalence. J Rheumatol 2003;30(8):1835–40.

[4] Neumann L, Buskila D. Epidemiology of fibromyalgia. Curr Pain Headache Rep 2003;7(5): 362–8.

[5] Lindell L, Bergman S, Petersson IF, et al. Prevalence of fibromyalgia and chronic widespread pain. Scand J Prim Health Care 2000;18(3): 149–53.

[6] Gran JT. The epidemiology of chronic generalized musculoskeletal pain. Best Pract Res Clin Rheumatol 2003;17(4):547–61.

[7] Makela M, Heliovaara M. Prevalence of primary fibromyalgia in the Finnish population. BMJ 1991;303(6796):216–9.

[8] Forseth KO, Gran JT. The prevalence of fibromyalgia among women aged 20-49 years in Arendal, Norway. Scand J Rheumatol 1992;21(2): 74–8.

[9] Prescott E, Kjoller M, Jacobsen S, et al. Fibromyalgia in the adult Danish population: I. A prevalence study. Scand J Rheumatol 1993; 22(5):233–7.

[10] Wolfe F, Hawley DJ. Fibromyalgia in the adult Danish population. Scand J Rheumatol 1994; 23(1):55–6.

[11] Hartz A, Kirchdoerfer E. Undetected fibrositis in primary care practice. J Fam Pract 1987;25(4): 365–9.

[12] Wolfe F, Cathey MA. Prevalence of primary and secondary fibrositis. J Rheumatol 1983;10(6): 965–8.

[13] Bengtsson A, Henriksson KG, Jorfeldt L, et al. Primary fibromyalgia. A clinical and laboratory study of 55 patients. Scand J Rheumatol 1986; 15(3):340–7.

[14] Cathey MA, Wolfe F, Kleinheksel SM. Functional ability and work status in patients with fibromyalgia. The burden of musculoskeletal diseases in the general population of Spain: results from a national survey. Arthritis Care Res 1988;60(1):85–98.

[15] Robinson RL, Birnbaum HG, Morley MA, et al. Economic cost and epidemiological characteristics of patients with fibromyalgia claims. J Rheumatol 2003;30(6):1318–25.

[16] Cathey MA, Wolfe F, Kleinheksel SM, et al. Socioeconomic impact of fibrositis. A study of 81 patients with primary fibrositis. Am J Med 1986;81(3A):78–84.

[17] Wolfe F, Smythe HA, Yunus MB, et al. The American College of Rheumatology 1990 criteria for the classification of fibromyalgia. Report of the Multicenter Criteria Committee. Arthritis Rheum 1990;33(2):160–72.

[18] de Girolamo G. Epidemiology and social costs of low back pain and fibromyalgia. Clin J Pain 1991;7(Suppl 1):S1–7.

[19] Carmona L, Ballina J, Gabriel R, et al. The burden of musculoskeletal diseases in the general population of Spain: results from a national survey. Ann Rheum Dis 2001;60(11):1040–5.

[20] Moldofsky H. Sleep and pain. Sleep Med Rev 2001;5(5):385–96.

[21] Nicassio PM, Moxham EG, Schuman CE, et al. The contribution of pain, reported sleep quality, and depressive symptoms to fatigue in fibromyalgia. Pain 2002;100(3):271–9.

[22] Korszun A. Sleep and circadian rhythm disorders in fibromyalgia. Curr Rheumatol Rep 2000; 2(2):124–30.

[23] Moldofsky H. Sleep and fibrositis syndrome. Rheum Dis Clin North Am 1989;15(1):91–103.

[24] Jennum P, Drewes AM, Andreasen A, et al. Sleep and other symptoms in primary fibromyalgia and in healthy controls. J Rheumatol 1993; 20(10):1756–9.

[25] Moldofsky H. Sleep and musculoskeletal pain. Am J Med 1986;81(3A):85–9.

[26] Branco J, Atalaia A, Paiva T. Sleep cycles and alpha-delta sleep in fibromyalgia syndrome. J Rheumatol 1994;21(6):1113–7.

[27] Moldofsky H, Scarisbrick P, England R, et al. Musculosketal symptoms and non-REM sleep disturbance in patients with "fibrositis syndrome" and healthy subjects. Psychosom Med 1975;37(4):341–51.

[28] Shapiro CM, Devins GM, Hussain MR. ABC of sleep disorders. Sleep problems in patients with medical illness. BMJ 1993;306(6891):1532–5.

[29] Perlis ML, Giles DE, Bootzin RR, et al. Alpha sleep and information processing, perception of sleep, pain, and arousability in fibromyalgia. Int J Neurosci 1997;89(3–4):265–80.

[30] Drewes AM, Nielsen KD, Taagholt SJ, et al. Sleep intensity in fibromyalgia: focus on the microstructure of the sleep process. Br J Rheumatol 1995;34(7):629–35.

[31] Shuer ML. Fibromyalgia: symptom constellation and potential therapeutic options. Endocrine 2003;22(1):67–76.

[32] Affleck G, Urrows S, Tennen H, et al. Sequential daily relations of sleep, pain intensity, and attention to pain among women with fibromyalgia. Pain 1996;68(2–3):363–8.

[33] Moldofsky H, Lue FA. The relationship of alpha and delta EEG frequencies to pain and mood in 'fibrositis' patients treated with chlorpromazine and L-tryptophan. Electroencephalogr Clin Neurophysiol 1980;50(1–2):71–80.

[34] Haythornthwaite JA, Hegel MT, Kerns RD. Development of a sleep diary for chronic pain patients. J Pain Symptom Manage 1991;6(2): 65–72.

[35] Pilowsky I, Crettenden I, Townley M. Sleep disturbance in pain clinic patients. Pain 1985; 23(1):27–33.

[36] Smythe HA. Does modification of sleep patterns cure fibrositis? Br J Rheumatol 1988; 27(6):449.

[37] Osorio CD, Gallinaro AL, Lorenzi-Filho G, et al. Sleep quality in patients with fibromyalgia using the Pittsburgh Sleep Quality Index. J Rheumatol 2006;33(9):1863–5.

[38] Agargun MY, Tekeoglu I, Gunes A, et al. Sleep quality and pain threshold in patients with fibromyalgia. Compr Psychiatry 1999;40(3): 226–8.

[39] Ohayon MM. Prevalence and correlates of nonrestorative sleep complaints. Arch Intern Med 2005;165(1):35–41.

[40] Korszun A, Young EA, Engleberg NC, et al. Use of actigraphy for monitoring sleep and activity levels in patients with fibromyalgia and depression. J Psychosom Res 2002;52(6):439–43.

[41] Harding SM. Sleep in fibromyalgia patients: subjective and objective findings. Am J Med Sci 1998;315(6):367–76.

[42] Sarzi-Puttini P, Rizzi M, Andreoli A, et al. Hypersomnolence in fibromyalgia syndrome. Clin Exp Rheumatol 2002;20(1):69–72.

[43] Hauri P, Hawkins DR. Alpha-delta sleep. Electroencephalogr Clin Neurophysiol 1973;34(3): 233–7.

[44] Roizenblatt S, Moldofsky H, Benedito-Silva AA, et al. Alpha sleep characteristics in fibromyalgia. Arthritis Rheum 2001;44(1):222–30.

[45] Mahowald ML, Mahowald MW. Nighttime sleep and daytime functioning (sleepiness and fatigue) in less well-defined chronic rheumatic diseases with particular reference to the 'alpha-delta NREM sleep anomaly'. Sleep Med 2000;1(3):195–207.

[46] Rains JC, Penzien DB. Sleep and chronic pain: challenges to the alpha-EEG sleep pattern as a pain specific sleep anomaly. J Psychosom Res 2003;54(1):77–83.

[47] Harding S, Lee-Chiong TL. Sleep in fibromyalgia and chronic pain. In: Lee-Chiong TL, editor. Sleep: a comprehensive handbook. Hoboken (NJ): Wiley-Liss; 2006. p. 759–66.

[48] Smith MT, Haythornthwaite JA. How do sleep disturbance and chronic pain inter-relate? Insights from the longitudinal and cognitive-behavioral clinical trials literature. Sleep Med Rev 2004;8(2):119–32.

[49] Moldofsky H. Management of sleep disorders in fibromyalgia. Rheum Dis Clin North Am 2002;28(2):353–65.

[50] Gold AR, Dipalo F, Gold MS, et al. Inspiratory airflow dynamics during sleep in women with fibromyalgia. Sleep 2004;27(3): 459–66.

[51] Yunus MB, Aldag JC. Restless legs syndrome and leg cramps in fibromyalgia syndrome: a controlled study. BMJ 1996;312(7042):1339.

[52] Hench P, Cohen R, Mitler M. Fibromyalgia: effects of amitriptyline, temazepam, and placebo on pain and sleep. Arthritis Rheum 1989; 32(Suppl):S47.

[53] Drewes AM, Andreasen A, Jennum P, et al. Zopiclone in the treatment of sleep abnormalities in fibromyalgia. Scand J Rheumatol 1991;20(4): 288–93.

[54] Gronblad M, Nykanen J, Konttinen Y, et al. Effect of zopiclone on sleep quality, morning stiffness, widespread tenderness and pain and general discomfort in primary fibromyalgia patients. A double-blind randomized trial. Clin Rheumatol 1993;12(2):186–91.

[55] Moldofsky H, Lue FA, Mously C, et al. The effect of zolpidem in patients with fibromyalgia: a dose ranging, double blind, placebo controlled, modified crossover study. J Rheumatol 1996;23(3):529–33.

[56] Van Cauter E, Plat L, Scharf MB, et al. Simultaneous stimulation of slow-wave sleep and growth hormone secretion by gamma-hydroxybutyrate in normal young Men. J Clin Invest 1997;100(3):745–53.

[57] Scharf MB, Baumann M, Berkowitz DV. The effects of sodium oxybate on clinical symptoms and sleep patterns in patients with fibromyalgia. J Rheumatol 2003;30(5):1070–4.

[58] Wikner J, Hirsch U, Wetterberg L, et al. Fibromyalgia—a syndrome associated with decreased nocturnal melatonin secretion. Clin Endocrinol (Oxf) 1998;49(2):179–83.

[59] Press J, Phillip M, Neumann L, et al. Normal melatonin levels in patients with fibromyalgia syndrome. J Rheumatol 1998;25(3):551–5.

[60] Korszun A, Sackett-Lundeen L, Papadopoulos E, et al. Melatonin levels in women with fibromyalgia and chronic fatigue syndrome. J Rheumatol 1999;26(12):2675–80.

[61] Acuna-Castroviejo D, Escames G, Reiter RJ. Melatonin therapy in fibromyalgia. J Pineal Res 2006;40(1):98–9.

[62] Citera G, Arias MA, Maldonado-Cocco JA, et al. The effect of melatonin in patients with fibromyalgia: a pilot study. Clin Rheumatol 2000; 19(1):9–13.

[63] Geenen R, Jacobs JW, Bijlsma JW. Evaluation and management of endocrine dysfunction in fibromyalgia. Rheum Dis Clin North Am 2002;28(2):389–404.

[64] Klerman EB, Goldenberg DL, Brown EN, et al. Circadian rhythms of women with fibromyalgia. J Clin Endocrinol Metab 2001;86(3): 1034–9.

[65] Rao SG, Bennett RM. Pharmacological therapies in fibromyalgia. Best Pract Res Clin Rheumatol 2003;17(4):611–27.

[66] Arnold LM, Keck PE Jr, Welge JA. Antidepressant treatment of fibromyalgia. A meta-analysis and review. Psychosomatics 2000;41(2):104–13.

[67] O'Malley PG, Balden E, Tomkins G, et al. Treatment of fibromyalgia with antidepressants:

a meta-analysis. J Gen Intern Med 2000;15(9): 659–66.

[68] Goldenberg D, Mayskiy M, Mossey C, et al. A randomized, double-blind crossover trial of fluoxetine and amitriptyline in the treatment of fibromyalgia. Arthritis Rheum 1996;39(11): 1852–9.

[69] Carette S, Oakson G, Guimont C, et al. Sleep electroencephalography and the clinical response to amitriptyline in patients with fibromyalgia. Arthritis Rheum 1995;38(9):1211–7.

[70] Branco J, Martini A, Paiva T. Treatment of sleep abnormalities and clinical complaints in fibromyalgia with trazodone. Arthritis Rheum 1996; 39(Suppl):S91.

[71] Barkhuizen A. Pharmacologic treatment of fibromyalgia. Curr Pain Headache Rep 2001; 5(4):351–8.

[72] Reynolds WJ, Moldofsky H, Saskin P, et al. The effects of cyclobenzaprine on sleep physiology and symptoms in patients with fibromyalgia. J Rheumatol 1991;18(3):452–4.

[73] Carette S, Bell MJ, Reynolds WJ, et al. Comparison of amitriptyline, cyclobenzaprine, and placebo in the treatment of fibromyalgia. A randomized, double-blind clinical trial. Arthritis Rheum 1994;37(1):32–40.

[74] Santandrea S, Montrone F, Sarzi-Puttini P, et al. A double-blind crossover study of two cyclobenzaprine regimens in primary fibromyalgia syndrome. J Int Med Res 1993;21(2): 74–80.

[75] Fossaluzza V, De Vita S. Combined therapy with cyclobenzaprine and ibuprofen in primary fibromyalgia syndrome. Int J Clin Pharmacol Res 1992;12(2):99–102.

[76] Bennett RM, Gatter RA, Campbell SM, et al. A comparison of cyclobenzaprine and placebo in the management of fibrositis. A double-blind controlled study. Arthritis Rheum 1988;31(12): 1535–42.

[77] Tofferi JK, Jackson JL, O'Malley PG. Treatment of fibromyalgia with cyclobenzaprine: a meta-analysis. Arthritis Rheum 2004;51(1):9–13.

[78] Hindmarch I, Dawson J, Stanley N. A double-blind study in healthy volunteers to assess the effects on sleep of pregabalin compared with alprazolam and placebo. Sleep 2005;28(2): 187–93.

[79] Crofford LJ, Rowbotham MC, Mease PJ, et al. Pregabalin for the treatment of fibromyalgia syndrome: results of a randomized, double-blind, placebo-controlled trial. Arthritis Rheum 2005;52(4):1264–73.

[80] Spath M. Current experience with 5-HT3 receptor antagonists in fibromyalgia. Rheum Dis Clin North Am 2002;28(2):319–28.

[81] Tolk J, Kohnen R, Muller W. Intravenous treatment of fibromyalgia with the 5-HT3 receptor antagonist tropisetron in a rheumatological practice. Scand J Rheumatol Suppl 2004; 33(119):72–5.

[82] Papadopoulos IA, Georgiou PE, Katsimbri PP, et al. Treatment of fibromyalgia with tropisetron, a 5HT3 serotonin antagonist: a pilot study. Clin Rheumatol 2000;19(1):6–8.

[83] Farber L, Stratz TH, Bruckle W, et al. Short-term treatment of primary fibromyalgia with the 5-HT3-receptor antagonist tropisetron. Results of a randomized, double-blind, placebo-controlled multicenter trial in 418 patients. Int J Clin Pharmacol Res 2001;21(1):1–13.

[84] Kohnen R, Farber L, Spath M. The assessment of vegetative and functional symptoms in fibromyalgia patients: the tropisetron experience. Scand J Rheumatol Suppl 2004;33(119):67–71.

[85] Hidalgo J, Rico-Villademoros F, Calandre EP. An open-label study of quetiapine in the treatment of fibromyalgia. Prog Neuropsychopharmacol Biol Psychiatry 2007;31(1):71–7.

[86] Palangio M, Flores JA, Joyal SV. Treatment of fibromyalgia with sibutramine hydrochloride monohydrate: comment on the article by Goldenberg et al. Arthritis Rheum 2002;46(9): 2545–6 [author reply: 2546].

[87] Kurtais Y, Kutlay S, Ergin S. Exercise and cognitive-behavioural treatment in fibromyalgia syndrome. Curr Pharm Des 2006;12(1): 37–45.

[88] Goldenberg D, Kaplan K, Nadeau M, et al. A controlled study of a stress-reduction, cognitive-behavioral treatment program in fibromyalgia. J Muscoskel Pain 1994;2:53–66.

[89] Stepanski EJ, Rybarczyk B. Emerging research on the treatment and etiology of secondary or comorbid insomnia. Sleep Med Rev 2006; 10(1):7–18.

[90] Morin C. Psychological and behavioral treatments for primary insomnia. In: Kryger MH, Roth T, Dement WC, editors. Principles and practice of sleep medicine. 4th edition. Philadelphia: Elsevier/Saunders; 2005. p. 726–37.

[91] Edinger JD, Wohlgemuth WK, Krystal AD, et al. Behavioral insomnia therapy for fibromyalgia patients: a randomized clinical trial. Arch Intern Med 2005;165(21):2527–35.

[92] Burckhardt CS. Nonpharmacologic management strategies in fibromyalgia. Rheum Dis Clin North Am 2002;28(2):291–304.

[93] Busch A, Schachter CL, Peloso PM, et al. Exercise for treating fibromyalgia syndrome. Cochrane Database Syst Rev 2002;3:CD003786.

[94] Altan L, Bingol U, Aykac M, et al. Investigation of the effects of pool-based exercise on fibromyalgia syndrome. Rheumatol Int 2004;24(5): 272–7.

[95] Wigers SH, Stiles TC, Vogel PA. Effects of aerobic exercise versus stress management treatment in fibromyalgia. A 4.5 year prospective study. Scand J Rheumatol 1996;25(2):77–86.

[96] Morris CR, Bowen L, Morris AJ. Integrative therapy for fibromyalgia: possible strategies for an individualized treatment program. South Med J 2005;98(2):177–84.

[97] Edwards A, Blackburn L, Christie S, et al. Food supplements in the treatment of primary fibromyalgia: a double-blind, crossover trial of anthocyanidins and placebo. J Nutr Environ Med 2000;10:189–99.

[98] Kaartinen K, Lammi K, Hypen M, et al. Vegan diet alleviates fibromyalgia symptoms. Scand J Rheumatol 2000;29(5):308–13.

[99] Puttini PS, Caruso I. Primary fibromyalgia syndrome and 5-hydroxy-L-tryptophan: a 90-day open study. J Int Med Res 1992;20(2):182–9.

[100] Caruso I, Sarzi Puttini P, Cazzola M, et al. Double-blind study of 5-hydroxytryptophan versus placebo in the treatment of primary fibromyalgia syndrome. J Int Med Res 1990;18(3):201–9.

[101] Pioro-Boisset M, Esdaile JM, Fitzcharles MA. Alternative medicine use in fibromyalgia syndrome. Arthritis Care Res 1996;9(1):13–7.

[102] Haanen HC, Hoenderdos HT, van Romunde LK, et al. Controlled trial of hypnotherapy in the treatment of refractory fibromyalgia. J Rheumatol 1991;18(1):72–5.

[103] Holmer M. The effects of yoga on symptoms and psychosocial adjustment in fibromyalgia syndrome patients. Dissertation Abstracts International: Section B: The Sciences and Engineering 2004;65(5B):2630.

[104] Hains G, Hains F. A combined ischemic compression and spinal manipulation in the treatment of fibromyalgia: a preliminary estimate of dose and efficacy. J Manipulative Physiol Ther 2000;23(4):225–30.

[105] Crofford LJ, Appleton BE. Complementary and alternative therapies for fibromyalgia. Curr Rheumatol Rep 2001;3(2):147–56.

[106] Davies AE, Davey RW. Effect of homoeopathic treatment on fibrositis. BMJ 1989;299(6704):918.

[107] Deluze C, Bosia L, Zirbs A, et al. Electroacupuncture in fibromyalgia: results of a controlled trial. BMJ 1992;305(6864):1249–52.

[108] Mueller HH, Donaldson CC, Nelson DV, et al. Treatment of fibromyalgia incorporating EEG-driven stimulation: a clinical outcomes study. J Clin Psychol 2001;57(7):933–52.

[109] Gur A, Karakoc M, Nas K, et al. Effects of low power laser and low dose amitriptyline therapy on clinical symptoms and quality of life in fibromyalgia: a single-blind, placebo-controlled trial. Rheumatol Int 2002;22(5):188–93.

[110] Almeida TF, Roizenblatt S, Benedito-Silva AA, et al. The effect of combined therapy (ultrasound and interferential current) on pain and sleep in fibromyalgia. Pain 2003;104(3):665–72.

[111] Turk D, Sherman J. Treatment of patients with fibromyalgia syndrome. In: Turk D, Gatchel R, editors. Psychological approaches to pain management: a practitioner's handbook. 2nd edition. New York: Guilford Press; 2002. p. 390–416.

[112] Beltran R. The effects of a supervised group aerobic exercise program and a chronobiologically oriented treatment protocol on symptomatology and mood in women with fibromyalgia. Dissertation Abstracts International: Section B: The Sciences and Engineering. 2003;64(2-B):955.

[113] Singh BB, Berman BM, Hadhazy VA, et al. A pilot study of cognitive behavioral therapy in fibromyalgia. Altern Ther Health Med 1998;4(2):67–70.

[114] Parkinson W, Cott A, Adachi J, et al. Follow-up of interdisciplinary medical and behavioural treatment for fibromyalgia. Arthritis Rheum 1996;39(Suppl):S212.

[115] Edinger JD, Bonnet MH, Bootzin RR, et al. Derivation of research diagnostic criteria for insomnia: report of an American Academy of Sleep Medicine Work Group. Sleep 2004;27(8):1567–96.

SLEEP
MEDICINE
CLINICS

Sleep Med Clin 2 (2007) 41–50

Gastroesophageal Reflux During Sleep

Susan M. Harding, MD

- Esophageal function during wakefulness and sleep
  Esophageal function
  Esophageal function during sleep
- Sleep-related GER
- Extraesophageal manifestations of sleep-related GER
- Sleep-related GER and obstructive sleep apnea
- Diagnosis of sleep-related GER
- Management of sleep-related GER
- Summary
- Acknowledgment
- References

Gastroesophageal reflux (GER) is a condition whereby gastric contents traverse into the esophagus through the lower esophageal sphincter (LES). In the United States, 44% of adults report heartburn at least once a month, 14% of adults report heartburn at least weekly, and 7% have it daily [1,2]. Because obesity is one of the risk factors for developing GER, GER prevalence will likely increase [3,4]. Heartburn and regurgitation are the most common symptoms of GER; however, GER can be asymptomatic [1,2,5]. GER can lead to complications including decreased quality of life, erosive esophagitis, strictures, Barrett's esophagus, esophageal bleeding, and adenocarcinoma of the esophagus [1,2,6]. Extraesophageal manifestations of GER are noted in the larynx and lung. Gastroesophageal reflux is also a cause of chest pain [7].

Gastroesophageal reflux also occurs during sleep and can disrupt sleep, cause excessive daytime sleepiness, and is a potential comorbid factor in other primary sleep disorders, including obstructive sleep apnea [8–10]. This review will examine esophageal function during sleep, manifestations of sleep-related GER and discuss a diagnostic and treatment strategy.

Esophageal function during wakefulness and sleep

Esophageal function

Despite its simple function of propelling food from the mouth to the stomach, esophageal function is complex. At the proximal end lies the upper esophageal sphincter (UES)—a high-pressure zone that includes the cricopharyngeal muscle. The esophageal body in adults extends 18 to 22 cm from the UES. From its proximal origin, the esophageal body is composed of striated muscle in the first 4 cm followed by a mixture of striated muscle and smooth muscle for the next 4 to 8 cm, ending exclusively with smooth muscle at its distal point. At the distal end of the esophagus is the LES [11]. The LES is a 2- to 4-cm high-pressure zone

This work is supported by NIH-NHLBI grant RO1-HL75614-01; S.M.H. has also received previous consultancy fees from AstraZeneca LP.
UAB Sleep-Wake Disorders Center, Division of Pulmonary, Allergy & Critical Care Medicine, University of Alabama at Birmingham, 1900 University Boulevard, THT Room 215, 1530 3rd Avenue South, Birmingham, AL 35294, USA
E-mail address: sharding@uab.edu

doi:10.1016/j.jsmc.2006.11.007

consisting of an intrinsic muscular layer (intrinsic LES) and the diaphragmatic crura. The intrinsic LES has cholinergic innervation and the diaphragmatic crura have bilateral phrenic nerve innervation. The intrinsic LES and the crural diaphragm are anchored to each other by the phrenoesophageal ligament. The intrinsic LES maintains a tonic contraction and relaxes with deglutination or esophageal distention. The diaphragmatic crura produces spike-like increases in LES pressure during inspiration and relaxes with esophageal distention as well as vomiting. Both the intrinsic LES and the diaphragmatic crura make up the LES antireflux barrier [11].

The esophagus has three types of contractions—primary, secondary, and nonperistaltic. Primary esophageal peristaltic contractions occur with swallowing, last 2 to 3 seconds, and their amplitude ensures an adequate push to propel the solid or liquid bolus. Secondary peristaltic contractions are localized to the esophagus and are not associated with swallowing or UES relaxation. Secondary peristaltic contractions remove leftover residue in the esophagus. Nonperistaltic contractions break up food in the esophagus.

On the other hand, transient LES relaxations (TLESRs) are LES relaxations that occur without swallowing. They occur with belching, vomiting, and rumination, and are vagally mediated [12]. Transient LES relaxations are the major mechanisms of GER and are responsible for 63% to 74% of GER episodes. Triggers of TLESRs include gastric distention and pharyngeal intubation. Patients with GER have a higher frequency of TLESRs compared with control subjects [12].

Promoting factors for GER include increased gastric acid secretion, delayed gastric emptying, and increased gastric pressure. Large pleural-abdominal pressure gradients, obesity, esophageal dysmotility, LES hypotension, and hiatal hernia also predispose to GER development. Most often the refluxate is acidic in nature; however, nonacid reflux can also lead to esophageal damage [13].

When GER episodes occur, esophageal acid clearance mechanisms come into play [14]. Salivation stimulates swallowing, resulting in primary peristalsis. Usually, most of the refluxate is cleared within the first two to three swallows and the resulting primary peristaltic contractions. Swallows also deliver bicarbonate-containing saliva, which neutralizes the acid refluxate.

Esophageal function during sleep

There are many physiologic changes that occur during sleep that are listed in Box 1. Esophageal acid clearance is markedly delayed, creating vulnerability to the complications of GER. Also, the

---

Box 1: GER physiology: sleep effects

- Basal gastric acid secretion peaks between 8 PM and 1 AM
- Delayed gastric emptying
- No salivary secretion
- No swallowing during stable sleep
- Upper esophageal sphincter pressure (UES) drops from 44 to 10 mm Hg
- UES reflex persists during REM sleep
- Lower esophageal sphincter (LES) pressure does not change
- Transient LES relaxations do not occur during stable sleep
- Esophageal acid clearance is markedly delayed during sleep and requires arousal for clearance
- Esophageal acid migrates proximal

---

circadian rhythm of basal gastric acid secretion peaks between 8 PM and 1 AM [15]. Sleep also disrupts gastromyoelectric function, resulting in delayed gastric emptying, further predisposing to GER [16].

Sleep also decreases UES pressure. With sleep onset, UES pressure drops from 44 to 10 mm Hg, thus predisposing to aspiration if proximal migration of the refluxate occurs [17]. The UES, along with the UES reflex, protects the upper airway and prevents aspiration. Interestingly, the volume required to trigger the UES reflex is lower during REM sleep despite generalized UES hypotonia [18]. Lower esophageal sphincter pressure does not change significantly during sleep.

Sleep increases the vagal threshold for triggering TLESRs. Usually, TLESRs are confined to arousals and do not occur during stable sleep. However, if GER does occur during sleep, esophageal acid clearance is markedly delayed because of multiple events [19]. First, swallowing is almost nonexistent during stable sleep and occurs primarily during brief arousals [19]. Also, salivary secretion is not measurable during stable sleep, impairing acid neutralization [20]. Orr and colleagues [19] noted that 15 mL of 0.1 molar NaCl was cleared within 6 minutes during wakefulness; however, during sleep it took up to 25 minutes to clear. Esophageal acid clearance occurred during brief arousals. Sleep also prolongs the latency period between esophageal acid exposure and the timing of the first swallow. Sleep facilitates proximal acid migration and thus further predisposes to aspiration [21]. During wake time, GER events tend to be frequent but brief, whereas GER events that occur during sleep time are comparatively less frequent, but last significantly longer because of prolonged esophageal acid clearance times.

Furthermore, behavioral practices can predispose to sleep-related GER. Eating within 2 hours of sleep can predispose to sleep-related GER. In 2001 consecutive subjects undergoing esophageal pH testing, GER during sleep was more frequent during the first half of the sleep period compared with the second half of the sleep period. Subjects eating a meal within 2 hours of sleep onset were 2.46 times more likely to develop GER during sleep time compared with subjects who did not eat within 2 hours of sleep onset [22]. Sleeping in the right lateral decubitus position is also associated with higher esophageal acid contact times and longer esophageal clearance times compared with the other sleep positions. The left lateral decubitus position is the preferred sleep position for GER patients because GER events are least likely to occur in this position [23].

Sleep-related GER

Sleep-related GER is considered a sleep disorder and is more common than clinically recognized [24]. Box 2 reviews the potential consequences of sleep-related GER. Sleep-related GER symptoms are prevalent in GER patients. A national population-based telephone survey, conducted by the Gallup Organization [25], of 1000 people who suffer heartburn at least once weekly noted that nighttime heartburn was present in 79% of subjects, and of these, 75% reported that their heartburn affected their sleep. Sixty-three percent believed that heartburn negatively affected their ability to sleep well, and 40% believed that their sleep-related heartburn impaired their daytime functioning. Furthermore, of subjects who had sleep-related heartburn, 71% were taking over-the-counter medications where only 29% had adequate control of their sleep-related GER symptoms. More concerning is that only 49% of subjects taking prescribed medications for GER had adequate control of their sleep-related GER symptoms. So, in general, more than 75% of

patients with GER report sleep-related GER symptoms.

To better understand the prevalence of sleep-related GER in the general population, Fass and colleagues [26] examined heartburn during sleep time in the 15,314 subjects of the Sleep Heart Health Study. Twenty-five percent (3086) of subjects had heartburn during sleep time. Strong predictors for sleep-related GER in multivariate models include higher body mass index, more carbonated drink consumption, snoring, sleepiness (Epworth Sleepiness Scale), insomnia, use of benzodiazepines, hypertension, and asthma. This study confirms that heartburn occurring during sleep time more than once a week is common and is associated with daytime sleepiness and insomnia [26].

There are many consequences of sleep-related GER. As noted in the epidemiology studies, patients have insomnia, sleep disturbances, excessive daytime sleepiness, impaired daytime functioning, and impaired quality of life. Recent placebo-controlled trials for treatment of sleep-related GER show that many of these consequences improve with aggressive GER therapy. A recent placebo-controlled study (esomeprazole 20 mg, 40 mg, or placebo for 4 weeks) assessed nighttime heartburn in 750 subjects with GER-related sleep disturbances [27]. Secondary outcomes included resolution of sleep disturbance, sleep quality as measured by the Pittsburgh Sleep Quality Index, and work productivity. More than 50% of the esomeprazole-treated subjects had resolution of nighttime heartburn compared with 13% of the placebo group. At baseline, 83% of subjects reported poor sleep quality—defined as a global Pittsburgh Sleep Quality Index score of greater than 5. By 4 weeks, 73% of the esomeprazole-treated subjects had resolution of their GER-associated sleep disturbance. Work productivity also improved in the esomeprazole-treated group. Both the 20-mg and 40-mg doses of esomeprazole improved sleep quality, increased the number of work hours, and improved work productivity [27].

Along with sleep-related heartburn, there is an increased risk of esophageal adenocarcinoma observed in patients with sleep-related GER [6]. In a case-controlled study, Lagergren [6] reported that the odds ratio for esophageal adenocarcinoma was 10.8 (95% confidence interval; 7.0 to 16.7) in subjects with heartburn, regurgitation, or both occurring at least once weekly during their sleep time. This may be partially explained by prolonged esophageal acid contact times during sleep as well as the greater likelihood of back-diffusion of hydrogen ions back into the esophageal mucosa [28]. Both back-diffusion of hydrogen ions and delayed

---

Box 2: Consequences of sleep-related GER

- Insomnia
- Sleep disturbance
- Impaired daytime functioning
- Excessive daytime sleepiness
- Impaired quality of life
- Erosive esophagitis
- Barrett's esophagus
- Adenocarcinoma of the esophagus
- Recurrent pneumonia and aspiration
- Nocturnal asthma
- Nocturnal laryngospasm

esophageal acid clearance predispose to erosive esophagitis, Barrett's esophagus, and potentially a greater risk for esophageal adenocarcinoma [29,30].

Extraesophageal manifestations of sleep-related GER

Sleep-related GER can also affect other organs, including the lungs and the larynx [9]. Potential extraesophageal consequences include recurrent pneumonia from aspiration, nocturnal asthma, and nocturnal laryngospasm. If esophageal acid enters the distal esophagus during sleep, it can migrate proximally to the level of the UES. With decreased UES pressure and altered protective reflexes that accompany sleep, subjects are predisposed to upper airway aspiration. This is most commonly seen in patients with underlying impairment of laryngeal protective reflexes, including dysphagia. Preliminary evidence indicates that sleep-related GER may lead to recurrent pneumonia and aspiration [31]. Also, microaspiration of esophageal contents is very common in normal individuals. In a nuclear medicine study, Ruth and colleagues [32] noted evidence of overnight aspiration in 38% of healthy control subjects using scintigraphic monitoring with technetium-99 isotope and sulfur colloid.

Perhaps the most studied extraesophageal manifestation of GER is asthma. Approximately 50% of asthmatic patients have GER and many epidemiological studies link the association between nighttime wheezing to GER. The European Respiratory Health Survey examined more than 2600 subjects, including 450 asthmatic patients. Subjects with GER were more likely to have nighttime wheezing, breathlessness, and cough compared with subjects without GER [33]. Asthma was more frequent in subjects with nocturnal GER compared with those without nocturnal GER (9% versus 4%, $P < .005$). A follow-up study (from year 5 to 10 including 16,191 participants) noted that nocturnal GER was independently associated with future asthma development [34].

In addition to epidemiological studies linking sleep-related GER with asthma, Sontag and colleagues [35] examined 261 asthmatic patients and 218 control subjects for nighttime heartburn. Twice as many asthmatic patients compared with control subjects had heartburn (98% versus 42%) [35]. Asthmatic patients were also more likely to eat before bedtime (60%) and these asthmatic patients were more likely to have nighttime GER and nighttime bronchospasm.

Esophageal and tracheal acid influence airway reactivity and peak expiratory flow rates during sleep. Monitoring both esophageal and tracheal pH in nocturnal asthmatic patients with GER, peak expiratory flow rates dropped 8 L/m when there was a drop in esophageal pH compared with 84 L/m when there was a drop in tracheal pH during sleep time [36]. Tracheal acid episodes were more likely to be associated with prolonged esophageal GER episodes along with awakenings and bronchospasm during the night [36]. Cuttitta and colleagues [37] evaluated spontaneous GER episodes and airway patency during the night in asthmatic patients with GER. Both long and short GER episodes were associated with increases in respiratory resistance compared with baseline. A multiple stepwise regression analysis revealed that the most important predictor of a change in lower respiratory resistance was the duration of esophageal acid exposure. These data collectively suggest that esophageal acid during sleep is able to elicit bronchoconstriction.

Furthermore, GER treatment can improve asthma symptoms during sleep time. A double-blind randomized placebo-controlled trial using esomeprazole 40 mg twice daily for 16 weeks in 770 asthmatic patients showed that esomeprazole improved peak expiratory flow rates in asthmatic patients with nighttime asthma and GER symptoms. This study provides further evidence that sleep-related GER can influence nighttime asthma, and that treatment has the potential to improve asthma during sleep [38].

Sleep-related GER may also cause laryngospasm, particularly if refluxate migrates into the upper airway. Patients with sleep-related laryngospasm have an abrupt interruption of their sleep accompanied by a feeling of acute suffocation and stridor. Thurnheer and colleagues [39] reported a case series of 10 patients with sleep-related laryngospasm. Nine of 10 patients had GER documented by esophageal pH testing of which 6 responded to GER therapy. Patients with sleep-related laryngospasm should be investigated for GER.

Sleep-related GER and obstructive sleep apnea

Obesity is a risk factor for both GER and obstructive sleep apnea (OSA), so correcting for this important confounding factor is important when trying to link the association between sleep-related GER and OSA. With this in mind, sleep-related GER is common in patients with OSA. In the European Community Respiratory Health Survey of 2001 young adults aged 20 to 44 years old, 5% of men and 2% of women snored nightly [40]. Reflux symptoms were associated with disrupted breathing (odds ratio 3.8; 95% confidence interval,

1.4-10) [40]. Another epidemiological study in the same database noted that young adults with nocturnal GER symptoms were more likely to have apnea compared with those without nocturnal GER ($P < .01$) [33]. Epidemiology studies do note a potential interaction between these two disease states.

In patients with OSA, sleep-related GER is quite common. Green and colleagues [41] prospectively examined 331 OSA patients. Significant sleep-related GER symptoms were found in 62% of subjects before continuous positive airway pressure (CPAP) therapy. CPAP-compliant patients had a 48% improvement in nocturnal GER symptoms ($P < .001$) with CPAP; however, noncompliant CPAP patients had no change in their sleep-related GER symptoms. There was a strong correlation between higher CPAP pressure requirements and improvement in nocturnal GER symptom scores. This study helped clarify the idea that CPAP may be a potential treatment option for difficult to treat sleep-related GER [41]. Another study noted that esophagitis was present in 80% of subjects with OSA and GER. Logistic regression analysis showed a positive correlation between esophagitis severity and the apnea-hypopnea index (AHI) ($P = .02$) [42].

To carefully examine a temporal association between OSA and GER, polysomnography combined with esophageal pH testing is required. Several small studies have attempted to note a temporal correlation between sleep-related GER events and respiratory events. Ing and colleagues examined 63 patients with OSA (AHI of >15) and 41 controls matched for age, body mass index (BMI), forced expiratory volume at one second (FEV_1), and alcohol use (AHI of <5 events an hour) [43]. Forty-seven percent of GER events had no temporal relationship with apneic events, whereas 11% of GER events were preceded within 1 minute of apneic events, 30% were followed by apneic events, and 12% occurred simultaneously. Fifty-three percent of respiratory events were unrelated to GER events and 56% of arousals were unrelated to GER episodes. They noted that OSA patients had more prolonged and more frequent GER episodes compared with control subjects, and that GER was temporally related to 50% of the arousals with apnea. Currently, the precise nature of the OSA-GER relationship remains unclear. Berg and colleagues [44] examined 14 consecutive suspected OSA subjects with polysomnography, esophageal pressure, and esophageal pH monitoring to examine if swings in pleural pressure correlated with GER events. Eighty-one percent of all GER events occurred simultaneously with respiratory events. There was no relationship between GER events and esophageal pressure swings or the AHI. The relationship between OSA and GER is more complex than what might be expected from simple passive mechanical considerations; for instance, the transdiaphragmatic pressure gradient. This study supports the notion that GER is not caused by OSA but that GER may be facilitated by it.

Two recent studies support the notion that OSA and sleep-related GER are not causally related [45,46]. Kim and colleagues [45] noted no relationship between OSA and GER symptoms, nor the severity of OSA. More definitive data were provided by Morse and colleagues [46] who examined 136 patients with suspected OSA with polysomnography, GER symptom checklist, and the Sleep Heart Health Study Questionnaire. Seventy-four of their subjects had OSA. Self-reported GER symptoms were unrelated to OSA severity, and OSA was not influenced by GER severity.

In conclusion, data show that there is a coexistence of OSA and sleep-related GER in many patients [47,48]. Potentially, respiratory events can cause arousals that can trigger TLESRs and promote GER; however, the interaction between respiratory events and GER is complex. Both diseases are common and share similar risk factors for development, including obesity. Both diseases disrupt sleep and sleep architecture. Future research may help clarify the association between OSA and sleep-related GER.

Diagnosis of sleep-related GER

Sleep-related GER can present in many ways. It can present with multiple awakenings, substernal burning and/or chest discomfort, indigestion, or heartburn [7,9]. Other symptoms include a sour or bitter taste in the mouth, regurgitation, water brash, coughing, or choking. Some patients may not have esophageal symptoms and present with excessive daytime sleepiness without an obvious cause, so polysomnography with esophageal pH testing may be required to establish the diagnosis. Some subjects present with only extraesophageal manifestations of GER such as waking up suddenly with laryngospasm, cough, or symptoms of bronchoconstriction, including wheezing. Occasionally patients notice regurgitated contents on their pillow in the morning without remembering waking up during the night. Some patients awaken multiple times during the night for unknown reasons.

Esophageal pH testing can be used to document sleep-related GER, especially in patients who do not have GER symptoms. Esophageal pH testing is done over a 24-hour period to increase the test's sensitivity and specificity, which approximates 90% [49,50]. Esophageal pH testing can be integrated with polysomnography so that esophageal acid can be correlated with sleep events, including arousals, apneas, and hypopneas, increased chin electromyogram (EMG) tone, periodic limb movements, dyspnea, and laryngospasm. By definition, GER events occur when the pH drops to less than 4. The distal esophageal pH probe is placed 5 cm above the LES. Manometric determination of the LES is the gold standard for esophageal pH probe placement [49,50]. A reference lead is placed on the anterior chest wall and the esophageal pH probe is then connected to a portable data acquisition device that has an event marker that the patient pushes to note when symptoms occur. Patients also record meals and sleep time in a diary.

Esophageal pH testing can be integrated with polysomnographic monitoring. The esophageal pH reference lead needs to be recorded through an electrical isolation box before connecting to the polysomnograph's DC amplifier. The output needs to be in the range of 0 to 1 V. When examining GER events during polysomnography, make note of which events occur on a timeline axis when the esophageal pH drops below 4. Normal esophageal acid contact times have been determined for both the distal (5 cm above the LES) and the proximal (within 2 cm of the UES) probe [51]. Probe insertion by a gastroenterologist or esophageal pH laboratory personnel is recommended as the patient can then come to the sleep lab with the esophageal pH probe in place.

Newer technology monitors esophageal pH using a wireless system allowing for data collection for up to 48 hours [52]. The Bravo pH System (Medtronic, Shoreview, MN) eliminates the intranasal catheter. The pH telemetry capsule is deployed intraorally during endoscopy and is usually placed 6 cm above the esophageal squamocolumnar junction. During probe placement, a small amount of suction is applied to the capsule so that the capsule stays in contact with the esophageal mucosa. A 433-mHz frequency signal is transmitted from the probe to a receiver and the data are downloaded to a computer for analysis. This technique does not allow direct integration with polysomnography at this time [52].

Not all esophageal refluxate is acidic in nature, and esophageal impedance combined with pH monitoring can evaluate acidic and nonacidic GER events [13,53]. There are minimal data examining sleep-related nonacidic GER using esophageal impedance. The clinical importance of nonacidic GER is unknown.

Management of sleep-related GER

Management of sleep-related GER requires careful attention to chronotherapeutic principles to ensure adequate control of GER during sleep time. Management strategies include conservative or behavioral measures, medical therapy, and surgical therapy.

All patients should be educated about lifestyle modifications for sleep-related GER [54]. Specific measures include sleeping in the left lateral decubitus position [23]. Furthermore, sleeping on a wedge or elevating the head of the bed by 6 inches decreases esophageal acid contact times [55]. Refraining from eating within 2 hours of bedtime should also be implemented. Antacids and alginate acids are used to control acute GER symptoms [54]. If patients have OSA, nasal CPAP improves GER [41,43]. Occasionally nasal CPAP is used in patients with severe GER who are resistant to other therapies [43,56]. Other helpful behavioral therapies are summarized in Box 3. Recently, lifestyle measures for GER were evaluated using an evidence-based approach. Examining all of the potential measures as outlined in Box 3—head of bed elevation and left lateral decubitus position—improved overall esophageal acid contact times. Weight loss also improved both GER symptoms and esophageal acid contact times. The other interventions had minimal supporting data to support their use [57].

Medical therapy for sleep-related GER includes medications that inhibit gastric acid secretion (proton pump inhibitors and H_2 receptor antagonists) and prokinetic agents. Gastric acid secretion inhibitors were initially introduced in the 1970s with the

---

Box 3: GER management: conservative measures

- Abstain from eating within 2 hours of bedtime
- Avoid:
  Caffeine
  Nicotine
  Alcohol
  Chocolate
  Mints
  Carbonated beverages
  High-fat foods
  Tomato or citrus-based products
- Avoid (if possible) medications that can worsen GER:
  Anticholinergics
  Theophylline
  Prostaglandins
  Calcium channel blockers
  Alendronate
- Encourage weight loss if obese
- Elevate head of bed by 6 inches
- Sleep in left lateral decubitus position
- Consider nasal CPAP if obstructive sleep apnea (OSA) is present

H$_2$ receptor antagonists. All of the H$_2$ receptor antagonists have equal efficacy and include cimetidine (up to 800 mg twice a day or 400 mg four times a day), ranitidine (150 mg twice a day), nizatidine (100 mg twice a day), and famotidine (20 mg twice a day). H$_2$ receptor antagonists provide heartburn relief in approximately 50% of patients [54]. Proton pump inhibitors (PPIs) provide superior gastric acid suppression and have excellent safety profiles for more than 17 years. Box illustrates currently available PPIs with recommended doses. Proton pump inhibitors require an active gastric parietal cell for efficacy, thus all PPIs should be taken 30 to 60 minutes before meals. So, if patients have GER symptoms during sleep and you want to initiate PPI therapy, consider giving the PPI 30 to 60 minutes before eating the evening meal. There are minimal clinically relevant differences between PPIs. Omeprazole has the highest potential for drug interactions with warfarin, diazepam, and phenytoin. Lansoprazole alters theophylline levels, while pantoprazole has the lowest potential for drug interactions [58,59]. Rabeprazole may have a slightly quicker onset of action. None of the PPIs require dosing adjustments for hepatic or renal insufficiency.

Looking specifically at sleep-related GER symptoms, recent data show that 40 mg of esomeprazole provides better control than 20 mg of the same drug or 30 mg of lansoprazole [60]. A double-blind placebo-controlled randomized trial of subjects taking 20 mg or 40 mg of esomeprazole for 4 weeks showed that sleep-related GER symptoms were relieved in 53% of subjects taking 40 mg, and in 50% of subjects taking 20 mg of esomeprazole, compared with 12% of subjects on placebo. Another study showed comparable relief of sleep-related GER symptoms with 40 mg pantoprazole or 40 mg esomeprazole [61]. Comparison of PPIs across research studies is difficult. Most of these studies were funded by drug companies, so the data need to be interpreted with caution. Despite

potent gastric acid secretion inhibitors, many patients still have sleep-related GER symptoms while using them, and evidence shows that most patients have nocturnal gastric acid breakthrough while taking PPIs. Nocturnal gastric acid breakthrough occurs in 90% of control subjects using omeprazole 20 mg twice a day [62]. Initial studies showed that taking an H$_2$ receptor antagonist before bedtime improved nocturnal gastric acid breakthrough; however, this effect was lost after 7 days [63,64].

Gastroesophageal reflux is a motility disease, so it is not surprising that gastric acid secretion inhibitors do not totally control sleep-related GER. Prokinetic agents improve motility by increasing LES pressure, accelerating esophageal acid clearance mechanisms, and improving gastric emptying [54]. Metoclopramide 10 mg four times a day is the only Food and Drug Administration (FDA)-approved prokinetic agent available at this time in the United States. It has significant central nervous system (CNS) side effects in 20% to 50% of patients. Despite its limitations, it can be used in combination with gastric acid suppressive agents. Potential future medications for sleep-related GER include gamma-amino butyric acid (GABA) agonists, which inhibit TLESRs [65]. Baclofen, which has many side effects, is the only GABA agonist currently available [66]. Hopefully, newer agents will be developed and released within the next 5 years.

Surgical fundoplication is another potential treatment modality for sleep-related GER. Both open and laparoscopic Nissen fundoplication provides symptom resolution in 80% to 90% of GER patients [67]. Surgical complications include dysphagia, chest herniation, slipped fundoplication, a wrap that is too tight, and vagal nerve injury. Long-term outcomes of surgical fundoplication show that up to 62% of surgically treated patients still required GER medication postoperatively [68]. Surgical fundoplication can be considered in some patients. Endoscopic fundoplication is still considered experimental in sleep-related GER [69].

An overall management strategy for sleep-related GER is to implement conservative measures along with a PPI taken 30 to 60 minutes before dinner. If patients have continued sleep-related GER, then consider adding a prokinetic agent. Esophageal pH testing can also be used to document adequate control of esophageal acid during sleep while on GER therapy and to identify sleep-related GER in patients who do not have esophageal symptoms.

Box 4:   Proton pump inhibitors (PPIs)

PPI[a]	Dosage
Omeprazole	20 mg
Omeprazole	20 mg with HCO$_3$
Lansoprazole	30 mg
Pantoprazole	40 mg
Rabeprazole	20 mg
Esomeprazole	40 mg
S-tenatoprazole[b]	60 mg

[a] PPIs should be taken 30 to 60 minutes before a major meal.
[b] Not available in the United States.

Summary

During sleep, esophageal acid clearance mechanisms are impaired so that patients are vulnerable to sleep-related GER. Sleep-related GER is associated with GER symptoms as well as nocturnal arousals, disruption of sleep architecture, excessive daytime sleepiness, impaired quality of life, esophagitis, Barrett's esophagus, and esophageal carcinoma. Extraesophageal manifestations of sleep-related GER include asthma and laryngospasm. Diagnosis of sleep-related GER includes careful evaluation for GER symptoms, symptoms of extraesophageal GER, and esophageal pH testing alone or in combination with polysomnography. Treatment includes behavioral measures along with medical treatment using gastric acid secretion inhibitors, and prokinetic agents. Surgery is reserved for selected patients. Hopefully, future research will optimize GER identification, management, and treatment in patients with sleep-related GER.

Acknowledgment

I wish to recognize the editorial assistance of Arren M. Graf in the preparation of this publication.

References

[1] Locke G III, Talley NJ, Fett SL, et al. Prevalence and clinical spectrum of gastroesophageal reflux: a population-based study in Olmstead County, Minnesota. Gastroenterology 1997;112: 1448–56.

[2] Gallup Organization. A Gallup Organization National Survey: heartburn across America. Princeton (NJ): The Gallup Organization; 1988.

[3] Corley DA, Kubo A. Body mass index and gastroesophageal reflux disease: a systematic review and meta-analysis. Am J Gastroenterol 2006; 101:2619–28.

[4] Hampel H, Abraham NS, El-Serag HB. Meta-analysis: obesity and the risk for gastroesophageal reflux disease and its complications. Ann Intern Med 2005;143(3):199–211.

[5] Harding SM, Guzzo MR, Richter JE. The prevalence of gastroesophageal reflux in asthma patients without reflux symptoms. Am J Respir Crit Care Med 2000;162:34–9.

[6] Lagergren J, Bergstrom R, Lindgren A, et al. Symptomatic gastric esophageal reflux as a risk factor for esophageal adenocarcinoma. N Engl J Med 1998;345:825–31.

[7] Fass F, Achem SR, Harding S, et al. Supra-oesophageal manifestations of gastro-oesophageal reflux disease and the role of night-time gastro-oesophageal reflux. [review article]. Aliment Pharmacol Ther 2004;20(Suppl 9):26–38.

[8] Orr WC. Reflux events and sleep: are we vulnerable? Curr Gastroenterol Rep 2006;8:202–7.

[9] Sexton MW, Harding SM. Sleep-related reflux: a unique clinical challenge. J Respir Dis 2003; 24:398–406.

[10] Farup C, Kleinman L, Sloan S, et al. The impact of nocturnal symptoms associated with gastroesophageal reflux disease on health-related quality of life. Arch Intern Med 2001;161:45–7.

[11] Mittal RK, Balaban DH. The esophagogastric junction. N Engl J Med 1997;336:924–32.

[12] Mittal RK, Holloway RH, Penagini R, et al. Transient lower esophageal sphincter relaxation. Gastroenterology 1995;109:601–10.

[13] Zerbib F, Roman S, Ropert A, et al. Esophageal pH-impedance monitoring and symptom analysis in GERD: a study in patients off and on therapy. Am J Gastroenterol 2006;101(9):1956–63.

[14] Helm JF, Riedel DR, Teeter BC, et al. Determinants of esophageal acid clearance in normal subjects. Gastroenterology 1983;85:607–12.

[15] Moore JG. Circadian dynamics of gastric acid secretion and pharmacodynamics of H_2 receptor blockade. Ann N Y Acad Sci 1991;618:150–8.

[16] Elsenbruch S, Orr WC, Harnish MJ, et al. Disruption of normal gastric myoelectric functioning by sleep. Sleep 1999;22:453–8.

[17] Kahrilas PJ, Dodds WJ, Dent J, et al. Effect of sleep, spontaneous gastroesophageal reflux, and a meal on upper esophageal sphincter pressure in normal human volunteers. Gastroenterology 1987;92:466–71.

[18] Bajaj JS, Bajaj S, Sua KS, et al. Influence of sleep stages on esophago-upper esophageal sphincter contractile reflex and secondary esophageal peristalsis. Gastroenterology 2006;130:17–25.

[19] Orr WC, Johnson LF, Robinson MG. The effect of sleep on swallowing, esophageal peristalsis, and acid clearance. Gastroenterology 1984;86:814–9.

[20] Schneyer LH, Pigmar W, Heyahar L. Rate of flow on human parotid, sublingual, and submaxillary secretions during sleep. J Dent Res 1956;35: 109–14.

[21] Orr WC, Elsenbruch S, Harnish MJ, et al. Proximal migration of esophageal acid perfusions during waking and sleep. Am J Gastroenterol 2000; 95:37–42.

[22] Hila A, Castell DO. Nighttime reflux is primarily an early event. J Clin Gastroenterol 2005;39: 579–83.

[23] Khoury RM, Camacho-Lobato L, Katz PO, et al. Influence of spontaneous sleep positions on nighttime recumbent reflux in patients with gastroesophageal reflux disease. Am J Gastroenterol 1999;94:2069–73.

[24] American Academy of Sleep Medicine. International classification of sleep disorders diagnostic and coding manual. 2nd edition. Westchester (IL): American Academy of Sleep Medicine; 2005.

[25] Shaker R, Castell DO, Schoenfeld PS, et al. Nighttime heartburn is an under-appreciated clinical problem that impacts sleep and daytime function: the results of a Gallup Survey conducted on behalf of the American Gastroenterological Association. Am J Gastroenterol 2003;98: 1487–93.

[26] Fass R, Quan SF, O'Connor GT, et al. Predictors of heartburn during sleep in a large prospective cohort study. Chest 2005;127:1658–66.

[27] Johnson DA, Orr WC, Crawley JA, et al. Effect of esomeprazole on nighttime heartburn and sleep quality in patients with GERD: a randomized placebo-controlled trial. Am J Gastroenterol 2005;100:1914–22.

[28] Orr WC. Heartburn. Another danger at night? Chest 2005;127:1486–8.

[29] Adachi K, Fujishiro H, Katsube T, et al. Predominant nocturnal acid reflux in patients with Los Angeles grade D and C reflux esophagitis. J Gastroenterol Hepatol 2001;16:1191–6.

[30] Orr WC, Lackey C, Robinson MG, et al. Esophageal acid clearance during sleep in patients with Barrett's esophagus. Dig Dis Sci 1988;33:654–9.

[31] Pellegrini CA, DeMeester TR, Johnson LF, et al. Gastroesophageal reflux and pulmonary aspiration: incidence, functional abnormality, and results of surgical therapy. Surgery 1978;86:110–9.

[32] Ruth M, Carlsson S, Mansson I, et al. Scintigraphic detection of gastro-pulmonary aspiration in patients with respiratory disorders. Clin Physiol 1993;13:19–33.

[33] Gislason T, Janson C, Vermeire P, et al. Respiratory symptoms and nocturnal gastroesophageal reflux: a population-based study of young adults in three European countries. Chest 2002;121:158–63.

[34] Gunnbjornsdottir MI, Omenaas E, Gislason T, et al. Obesity and nocturnal gastro-esophageal reflux are related to onset of asthma and respiratory symptoms. Eur Respir J 2004;24:116–21.

[35] Sontag SJ, O'Connell S, Miller TQ, et al. Asthmatics have more nocturnal gasping and reflux symptoms than non-asthmatics, and they are related to bedtime eating. Am J Gastroenterol 2004;99:789–96.

[36] Jack CIA, Calverley PMA, Donnelly RJ, et al. Simultaneous tracheal and oesophageal pH measurement in asthmatic patients with gastro-oesophageal reflux. Thorax 1995;50:201–4.

[37] Cuttitta G, Cibella F, Visconti A. Spontaneous gastroesophageal reflux and airway patency during the night in adult asthmatics. Am J Respir Crit Care Med 2000;151:177–81.

[38] Kiljander TO, Harding SM, Field SK, et al. Effects of esomeprazole 40 mg twice daily on asthma. A randomized placebo-controlled trial. Am J Respir Crit Care Med 2006;173:1091–7.

[39] Thurnheer R, Henz S, Knoblauch A. Sleep-related laryngospasm. Eur Respir J 1997;10:2084–6.

[40] Janson C, Gislason TR, De Backer W, et al. Daytime sleepiness, snoring and gastro-oesophageal reflux amongst young adults in three European countries. J Intern Med 1995;237:277–85.

[41] Green BT, Broughton WA, O'Connor JB. Marked improvement in nocturnal gastroesophageal reflux in a large cohort of patients with obstructive sleep apnea. Arch Intern Med 2003;163:41–5.

[42] Demeter P, Visy KV, Magyar P. Correlation between severity of endoscopic findings and apnea-hypopnea index in patients with gastroesophageal reflux disease and obstructive sleep apnea. World J Gastroenterol 2005;14:839–41.

[43] Ing AJ, Ngu MC, Breslin AB. Obstructive sleep apnea and gastroesophageal reflux. Am J Med 2000;108(Suppl 4A):120S–5S.

[44] Berg S, Hoffstein V, Gislason T. Acidification of distal esophagus and sleep-related breathing disturbances. Chest 2004;125:2101–6.

[45] Kim H-N, Vorona RD, Winn MP, et al. Symptoms of gastro-oesophageal reflux disease and the severity of obstructive sleep apnoea syndrome are not related in sleep disorders center patients. Aliment Pharmacol Ther 2005;21:1127–33.

[46] Morse CA, Quan SF, Mays MZ, et al. Is there a relationship between obstructive sleep apnea and gastroesophageal reflux disease? Clin Gastroenterol Hepatol 2004;2:761–8.

[47] Senior BA, Khan M, Schwimmer C, et al. Gastroesophageal reflux and obstructive sleep apnea. Laryngoscope 2001;111:2144–6.

[48] Zanation AM, Senior BA. The relationship between extraesophageal reflux (EER) and obstructive sleep apnea (OSA). Sleep Med Rev 2005;9(6):453–8.

[49] Kahrilas PJ, Quigley EM. Clinical esophageal pH recording: a technical review for practice guideline development. Gastroenterology 1996;110:1982–96.

[50] Richter JE, editor. Esophageal pH monitoring: practical approach and clinical applications. 2nd edition. Baltimore (MD): Williams & Wilkins; 1997.

[51] Harding SM, Richter JE, Guzzo MR, et al. Asthma and gastroesophageal reflux: acid suppressive therapy improves asthma outcome. Am J Med 1996;100:395–405.

[52] Pandolfino JE, Richter JE, Ours T, et al. Ambulatory esophageal pH monitoring using a wireless system. Am J Gastroenterol 2003;98:740–9.

[53] Mainie I, Tutuian R, Shay S, et al. Acid and non-acid reflux in patients with persistent symptoms despite acid suppressive therapy: a multicenter study using combined ambulatory impedance-pH monitoring. Gut 2006;55:1398–402.

[54] DeVault KR, Castell DO. Updated guidelines for the diagnosis and treatment of gastroesophageal reflux disease: the Practice Parameters Committee of the American College of Gastroenterology. Am J Gastroenterol 1999;94:1434–42.

[55] Hamilton JW, Boisen RJ, Yamamoto DT, et al. Sleeping on a wedge diminishes exposure of the esophagus to refluxed acid. Dig Dis Sci 1988;33:518–22.

[56] Shoenut JP, Kerr P, Micflikier AB, et al. The effect of nasal CPAP on nocturnal reflux in patients with aperistaltic esophagus. Chest 1994;106(3):738–41.

[57] Kaltenbach T, Crockett S, Gerson LB. Are lifestyle measures effective in patients with gastroesophageal reflux disease? Arch Intern Med 2006;166: 963–71.

[58] Lundell L. Advances in treatment strategies for gastroesophageal reflux disease. In: Farthing MJG, Malfertheiner P, editors. Basic mechanisms of digestive diseases: the rationale for clinical management and prevention. Paris: John Libbey Eurotex; 2002. p. 13–22.

[59] Robinson M, Horn J. Clinical pharmacology of proton pump inhibitors: what the practicing physician needs to know. Drugs 2003;63(24): 2739–54.

[60] Orr WC. Therapeutic options in the treatment of nighttime gastroesophageal reflux. Digestion 2005;72:229–30.

[61] Orr WC. Night-time gastro-oesophageal reflux disease: prevalence, hazards, and management. Eur J Gastroenterol Hepatol 2005;17:113–20.

[62] Peghini PL, Katz PO, Bracy NA, et al. Nocturnal recovery of gastric acid secretion with twice-daily dosing of proton pump inhibitors. Am J Gastroenterol 1998;93:763–7.

[63] Fackler WK, Ours TM, Vaezi MF, et al. Long-term effect of H_2RA therapy on nocturnal acid break through. Gastroenterology 2002;122:625–32.

[64] Orr WC, Harnish MJ. The efficacy of omeprazole twice daily with supplemental H_2 blockade at bedtime in the suppression of nocturnal oesophageal and gastric acidity. Aliment Pharmacol Ther 2003;17:1553–8.

[65] Richter JE. New investigational therapies for gastroesophageal reflux disease. Thorac Surg Clin 2005;15(3):377–84.

[66] Vela MF, Tutuian R, Katz PO. Baclofen decreases acid and non-acid post-prandial gastro-oesophageal reflux measured by combined multichannel intraluminal impedance and pH. Aliment Pharmacol Ther 2003;17:243–51.

[67] Peters JH, Heimbucher J, Kauer WK, et al. Clinical and physiologic comparison of laparoscopic and open Nissen fundoplication. Am Coll Surg 1995;180:385–93.

[68] Spechler SJ, Lee E, Ahnen D, et al. Long-term outcome of medical and surgical therapies for gastroesophageal reflux disease: follow-up of a randomized controlled trial. JAMA 2001;285: 2331–8.

[69] Rothstein R, Filipi C, Caca K, et al. Endoscopic full-thickness placation for the treatment of gastroesophageal reflux disease: a randomized, sham-controlled trial. Gastroenterology 2006;131(3): 704–12.

SLEEP
MEDICINE
CLINICS

Sleep Med Clin 2 (2007) 51–58

ELSEVIER
SAUNDERS

HIV/AIDS

Steven Reid, MB, PhD[a,b,]*, Louise McGrath, RMN[a,c]

- HIV and AIDS
- Sleep architecture, immune function, and HIV infection
- Antiretroviral therapy
- Psychiatric disorders
- Alcohol and illicit drug use
- Pain
- Management of insomnia in HIV infection
- Pharmacological treatments
- Psychological treatments
- References

From the earliest clinical descriptions of the disease, insomnia has been recognized as a frequent complaint among patients with HIV [1,2]. Sleep disturbance is commonly reported at all stages of HIV infection and has been ascribed to a range of etiologic factors including the neurotropic effects of the HIV virus, antiretroviral therapy, HIV-related symptoms such as fatigue and night sweats, drug and alcohol use, and psychiatric illness [3].

Prevalence rates of insomnia in the general population range from 10% to 40%, but typically surveys show that sleep disturbance is more common among those with chronic medical illness [4–7]. The lack of large epidemiological studies makes it difficult to be certain about the prevalence of insomnia in HIV-positive populations and those studies available are limited by a lack of seronegative controls or small sample sizes. Many studies also fail to distinguish between insomnia as a symptom and as a disorder. However, the available evidence certainly indicates that sleep disturbance is commonly experienced in HIV and AIDS [8–10]. One cross-sectional survey used the Pittsburgh Sleep Quality Index to identify poor sleepers and found that 73% of a sample of outpatients had insomnia, requiring more than 1 hour to go to sleep compared with good sleepers, and on average sleeping for 2 hours less [11].

Persistent insomnia is associated with a number of adverse consequences including chronic fatigue, mood disturbance, cognitive impairment, impaired job performance, and increased health care use [5,12]. As well as having an impact on quality of life, it may also compromise treatment adherence, which is of particular importance in HIV infection [13].

HIV and AIDS

Currently an estimated 40 million people live with HIV/AIDS worldwide [14]. In 2005 there were 4.1 million new HIV infections and 3 million AIDS deaths [14]. Eighty-five percent of HIV infections are accounted for by heterosexual transmission [15]. Sub-Saharan Africa comprises the majority of infections but numbers are increasing rapidly in China and India [14]. In the United States it is estimated that over 1 million people are living with HIV [16]. African and Hispanic Americans are disproportionately affected with 70% of new infections occurring in these minority groups [16].

HIV disease begins with a latent infection, which over time (6 months to 15 years) progresses to AIDS. Early signs of HIV infection include flu-like symptoms, lymphadenopathy, poor appetite, and weight loss as well as insomnia [17]. The virus

[a] Department of Liaison Psychiatry, St Mary's Hospital, 20 South Wharf Road, London W2 1PD, UK
[b] Department of Psychological Medicine, Imperial College, Praed Street, London W2 1NY, UK
[c] Department of HIV Medicine, St Mary's Hospital, Praed Street, London W2 1NY, UK
* Corresponding author.
E-mail address: steve.reid@nhs.net (S. Reid).

doi:10.1016/j.jsmc.2006.11.009

attacks CD4+ T-lymphocytes, that are an integral component of the normal immune response, as well as microglial cells and macrophages that affect the central nervous system. After the primary infection the patient is often asymptomatic until the onset of overt immunodeficiency. The clinical course is highly variable and depends on the host immunology, viral properties, and genetic factors (Fig. 1). Progression to AIDS is predicted both by CD4+ count and plasma viral load. While the viral load determines the rate of destruction of the immune system, the CD4+ count is the primary marker of immunodeficiency and indicates the risk of opportunistic infections and other complications, particularly when the count is below 200 cells per microliter (Table 1) [14,17].

Although no current treatment eradicates HIV infection, antiretroviral treatment is the best option for viral suppression and has transformed the clinical course of the disease. Before the development of highly active antiretroviral therapy (HAART) the average life expectancy was 12 years but now, at least in the developed world, for many patients HIV infection is considered a chronic manageable illness [18,19]. The combination of several drugs that attack different parts of the replication cycle slows disease progression, partially restoring immune function and minimizing resistance (Table 2). Rigorous adherence to treatment is essential for maintaining suppression of the viral load. Partial or poor adherence can lead to the resumption of rapid viral replication and adherence rates of less than 95% are associated with the emergence of drug resistance, the development of opportunistic infections, and increased mortality [20,21].

Sleep architecture, immune function, and HIV infection

Early descriptive studies of seropositive patients using polysomnography indicated abnormalities of sleep pattern, suggesting that the neurotoxic HIV virus caused a progressive deterioration in sleep architecture [22]. Investigators reported a significant increase in slow wave sleep, particularly during the late sleep cycles [23–25]. There were also reports in otherwise asymptomatic individuals of an increased frequency but reduced duration of periods of rapid eye movement sleep [26]. These observations were linked with findings from animal studies to suggest a role for the cytokines, tumor necrosis factor (TNF-α) and interleukin-1 (IL-1) [22]. Elevated plasma levels of these immune mediators released by activated microglial and macrophages have been described in HIV-positive subjects [27]. A mechanism for disturbed sleep physiology in early HIV infection was suggested by evidence from trials of cancer chemotherapy where these cytokines were known to cause somnolence and fatigue [28]. However, these alterations of sleep architecture have not been found in subsequent controlled studies [29–31]. Examination of the effect of disease progression has also failed to establish a clear relationship, either when looking at CD4+ count or the categorical Centers for Disease Control and Prevention (CDC) stages of HIV infection [9–11,32–35]. The notable exception is late-stage, symptomatic illness (stage IV; CD4+ <200 cells/μL), which may be associated with manifest cerebral pathology [36,37]. In this group insomnia may be a direct consequence of an AIDS-defining

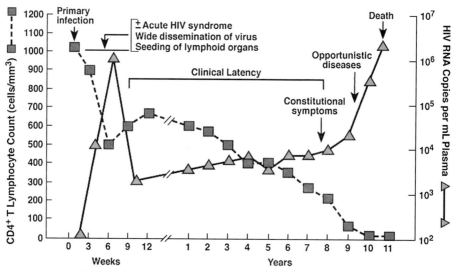

Fig. 1. Typical course of HIV infection. (*Adapted from* Pantaleo G, Graziosi C, Fauci AS. Mechanisms of Disease: the Immunopathogenesis of Human Immunodeficiency Virus Infection. New Engl J Med 1993;328:327–35.)

Table 1: Complications of HIV infection

Infectious complications	Noninfectious complications
Pneumococcal and other bacterial pneumonia	Persistent generalized lymphadenopathy
Pulmonary tuberculosis	Guillain-Barré syndrome
Herpes zoster	Aseptic meningitis
Thrush (oropharyngeal candidiasis)	Cervical carcinoma
Kaposi's sarcoma	B-cell lymphoma
Oral hairy leukoplakia	Anemia
Pneumocystis carinii pneumonia	Mononeuritis multiplex
Disseminated histoplasmosis	Idiopathic thrombocytopenic purpura
Coccidioidomycosis	Hodgkin's disease
Military/ extrapulmonary TB	Peripheral neuropathy
Progressive multifocal leukoencephalopathy	HIV-associated dementia
Disseminated herpes simplex	Cardiomyopathy
Toxoplasmosis	Vacuolar myelopathy
Cryptococcosis	Progressive polyradiculopathy
Microsporidiosis	Non-Hodgkin's lymphoma
Candida esophagitis	Central nervous system lymphoma
Disseminated cytomegalovirus	
Disseminated mycobacterium avium complex	

Table 2: Currently approved drugs for HIV

	Generic name	Common/ Trade name
Reverse transcriptase inhibitors		
Nucleoside/ Nucleotide (NRTIs)	Zidovudine	Retrovir
	Stavudine	Zerit
	Lamivudine	Epivir
	Didanosine	Videx
	Abacavir	Ziagen
	Emtricitabine	Emtriva
	Tenofivir DF	Viread
	Abacavir + Lamivudine	Epzicon or Kivexa
	Emtricitabine + Tenofivir DF	Truvada
	Lamivudine + Zidovudine	Combivir
	Lamivudine + Zidovudine + Abacavir	Trizivir
Nonnucleoside (NNRTIs)	Nevirapine	Viramune
	Delavirdine	Rescriptor
	Efavirenz	Sustiva
	Efavirenz + Tenofivir DF + Emtricitabine	Atripla
Protease inhibitors		
	Saquinavir	Invirase
	Ritonavir	Norvir
	Indinavir	Crixivan
	Nelfinavir	Viracept
	Darunavir	Prezista
	Atazanavir	Reyataz
	Fosamprenavir	Lexiva or Telzif
	Tipranavir	Aptivus
	Lopiniavir + Ritonavir	Kaletra
Entry inhibitors		
	Enfuvirtide	Fuzeon

illness and the abnormalities are similar to those found in other disorders affecting the central nervous system (CNS). The importance of CNS involvement is also indicated by the strength of association between insomnia and cognitive impairment [11]. At this stage of illness sleep becomes severely disrupted and studies have shown a marked reduction in slow wave sleep with increased fragmentation leading eventually to a complete destruction of the normal sleep structure [38–40].

Antiretroviral therapy

Although insomnia is commonly regarded as an adverse effect of antiretroviral drugs, in drug trials fewer than 10% of subjects complain of sleep disturbance [40]. However, these rates may underestimate the actual occurrence of adverse effects as few studies have systematically examined the risk of insomnia associated with antiretroviral drugs either individually or as a group [9,34]. To date, there is a lack of evidence to support a class effect of antiretroviral drugs [11,33]. Neuropsychiatric complications have been frequently reported with the non-nucleoside reverse transcriptase inhibitor efavirenz [41]. These include drowsiness, hallucinations, vivid dreams, and nightmares, and lead to drug discontinuation in 3% to 5% of treated individuals [41,42]. Severe depression, aggressive behavior, and psychotic symptoms may also occur [43,44]. As a consequence, efavirenz has been examined closely for its effect on sleep and a correlation with insomnia has been established with longer sleep latencies and shorter duration of deep sleep [45]. One study compared efavirenz with a protease inhibitor and found that 4 weeks after treatment initiation 35% of those prescribed efavirenz reported difficulty sleeping, compared with 4% in the protease inhibitor group [46]. Neuropsychiatric complications have also been reported with nevirapine, another non-nucleoside reverse transcriptase inhibitor [47]. A number of case reports describe nevirapine-induced insomnia and vivid dreams but the evidence for a consistent effect is limited [48]. What seems clear is that neuropsychiatric adverse effects are dose-dependent and that for the majority of patients the adverse effect profile declines in severity within 4 weeks of starting treatment [41].

HAART is also associated with the development of lipodystrophy in HIV-positive patients. This syndrome, most commonly occurring in patients receiving a combination regimen including protease inhibitors, is characterized by metabolic changes and notably, in particular weight gain, visceral adiposity, and peripheral lipoatrophy [49]. A prospective cohort study after initiation of therapy found a 17% prevalence rate after an 18-month follow-up period [50]. The accumulation of subcutaneous fat around the neck and pharynx may lead to obstructive sleep apnea, which usually manifests with complaints of snoring, daytime somnolence, and fatigue [51]. The diagnosis is confirmed by nocturnal polysomnography.

Psychiatric disorders

Psychological morbidity, and in particular depression, has a well-established association with insomnia [12,52]. Sleep disturbance is both a symptom and diagnostic criterion of both anxiety and depressive disorders, which complicates attempts to examine their relationship in the context of HIV infection. However, a systematic review of correlates of insomnia in HIV infection found that psychological morbidity was a major determinant of insomnia, more so than other factors such as disease progression or antiretroviral therapy [3]. This was demonstrated in two epidemiological studies [11,34]. One study followed 98 HIV-positive men over a period of 6 months and found that an increased score on the depression scale over that period of time predicted a worsening severity in insomnia. This association was not apparent with changes in CD4+ count or clinical disease progression [34]. The second study examined a mixed population of seropositive clinic attenders and found that among patients complaining of insomnia, both anxiety (65% versus 26%; $P < .01$) and

depression (41% versus 10%; $P < .01$) were more common [11]. These findings suggest that in a population of otherwise asymptomatic seropositive individuals, complaints of disturbed sleep are likely to be related to psychological morbidity. Similar findings have also been observed in studies of fatigue in HIV-positive populations [53]. Unsurprisingly, fatigue is a common and debilitating symptom in HIV infection, but as with insomnia, psychological distress seems more important than viral or immunological factors, or HAART.

Alcohol and illicit drug use

Given the association between intravenous drug use and HIV transmission it is not surprising that illicit drug use is common in people with HIV infection. In a large epidemiological study of psychiatric disorders and HIV disease in the United States, half of the sample receiving care for HIV reported illicit drug use in the previous 12 months, and 12% were positive for drug dependence [54]. Among a number of adverse health outcomes, substance misuse is associated with unsafe sexual behavior and may also affect treatment adherence. Despite the recognized disruptive effect of alcohol and illicit drugs on sleep, few studies have considered their effect in persons with HIV [3]. Many studies evaluating sleep in HIV populations have been limited by the exclusion of patients admitting to alcohol or recreational drug use. Furthermore, there may be underreporting of illicit drug use if patients fear they may be liable to criminal prosecution, making such information unreliable [10]. One study of 115 HIV-positive clinic attenders found a nonsignificant trend with 86% of 29 patients admitting to illicit drug use reporting chronic insomnia compared with 69% of nondrug users [11].

Pain

There are no published studies of the relationship between pain and insomnia in HIV infection but estimates of the prevalence of pain in this population range from 40% to 60%, increasing with severity of disease [55]. The 1991 General Social Survey by Statistics Canada showed that 44% of people with a painful disorder experience sleep problems and unsurprisingly, the greater the severity of pain, the higher the likelihood of having insomnia or unrefreshing sleep [56]. As with pain in other medical disorders it is both underestimated and undertreated [55,57,58]. Pain syndromes can be attributable to HIV infection itself or complications, such as Kaposi's sarcoma, opportunistic infections affecting the intestines or skin, arthritides, or myopathies [55]. Peripheral neuropathy, characterized by a sensation of burning and numbness in the affected extremity, affects up to 30% of seropositive people. Some antiretroviral drugs, notably nucleoside analog reverse transcriptase inhibitors (NRTIs), and prophylactic agents such as dapsone can also cause a toxic neuropathy [55].

Management of insomnia in HIV infection

Insomnia is common in HIV infection and has a significant impact on quality of life, yet it often remains untreated. As well as a problem with recognition, this may in part be because of uncertainty about management. There is a range of pharmacological and psychological treatments available for insomnia but there has been little evaluation of these treatments in people with HIV.

Thorough assessment is important, as insomnia is a heterogeneous complaint that may involve difficulties with sleep onset, frequent nocturnal or early morning wakening, or sleep that is nonrestorative [59]. It may also be transient, short-term, or chronic in duration. Short-term insomnia is mostly attributable to situational stressors and often responds to sleep hygiene measures (Box 1) [60]. A randomized controlled trial of caffeine withdrawal and abstinence found a 35% improvement in sleep in seropositive patients with a reduced intake [61]. Assessment should include a comprehensive medical and mental state examination to identify underlying physical and psychological factors (Box 2). Checking with the bed partner for snoring or pauses in breathing may indicate sleep apnea. Given that psychiatric disorders are often missed in medical settings, it is important that anxiety and depression are identified and treated. Daytime sleepiness should also be evaluated, with consideration given to driving and occupation-related hazards.

For patients with habitual or chronic insomnia, or in circumstances where causal factors such as pain are not fully manageable, simple sleep hygiene measures may be insufficient and detailed measurement using a sleep diary or log is recommended.

Box 1: Sleep hygiene measures

Maintain regular wake time
Avoid excessive time in bed
Avoid daytime naps
Exercise daily, finishing at least 4 hours before bedtime
Take a hot bath within 2 hours of bedtime
Drink a hot beverage without caffeine
Avoid caffeine, nicotine, and alcohol in the evening
Avoid large meals soon before bedtime
Develop a relaxing bedtime ritual

Box 2: Considerations in management of insomnia in asymptomatic HIV infection

Identify and treat anxiety and depression
Reduce caffeine, alcohol, and recreational drug use
Optimize pain management
Consider alternative antiretroviral drug if insomnia is a **persistent** adverse effect
Identify obstructive sleep apnea, particularly in presence of lipodystrophy

---

This will enable a calculation of sleep efficiency, which is the ratio of total sleep time to nocturnal time in bed. If sleep efficiency is less than 85% then specific treatments should be considered.

Pharmacological treatments

Clinical experience suggests that benzodiazepines and other hypnotics are the most frequently used treatment for insomnia in this population. While there is good evidence that in the short term (less than 4 weeks) benzodiazepines increase sleep duration, their effects on sleep efficiency particularly in the long term are uncertain [62,63]. Tolerance, rebound insomnia, prolonged sedation, and dependence are all recognized problems with both benzodiazepines and newer hypnotics (zopiclone, zaleplon). Therefore, it is recommended that, when used, hypnotics should be prescribed at the smallest effective dose for the shortest period of time. Importantly, protease inhibitors have been shown to raise the plasma levels of alprazolam, midazolam, and triazolam with the potential for respiratory depression, so these drugs should be avoided. Although based on limited evidence, low-dose antidepressants such as trazadone, amitriptyline, and nortriptyline are commonly used and may be helpful for selected patients.

Psychological treatments

A number of behavioral strategies have been shown to have a good effect in insomnia in the general population, and although yet to be evaluated in people with HIV they should be considered [64]. The most commonly used interventions are sleep hygiene education (vide supra), stimulus control, and sleep restriction [65,66]. They are also often used in combination. Stimulus control aims to redevelop the association between bedtime cues and sleep onset. The patients are instructed to go to bed only when sleepy and if unable to fall asleep within 20 minutes to get out of bed and leave the bedroom. They then return to bed only when sleepy and repeat the plan, arising at a regular time each morning. Sleep restriction may be helpful for patients with persistent, severe insomnia. With this technique patients are instructed to spend no more time in bed than they spent asleep the previous night. This restriction causes a mild sleep deprivation and time in bed is progressively increased as their sleep efficiency improves. If these measures are unsuccessful, evaluation by a sleep specialist should be considered, if available.

In conclusion, insomnia is a common problem in people living with HIV and has a significant impact on quality of life, with the potential to compromise optimal treatment. Among the many potential factors that may lead to sleep disturbance, psychological morbidity is a major determinant and complaints of insomnia should elicit detailed questioning about depression and anxiety.

References

[1] Herman P. Neurologic effects of HTLV-III infection in adults: an overview. Mt Sinai J Med 1986; 53:616–21.

[2] Norman SE, Resnick L, Cohn MA, et al. Sleep disturbances in HIV-seropositive patients. JAMA 1988; 260:7.

[3] Reid S, Dwyer J. Insomnia in HIV infection: a systematic review of prevalence, correlates, and management. Psychosom Med 2005;67:260–9.

[4] Mellinger GD, Balter MB, Uhlenhuth EH. Insomnia and its treatment: prevalence and correlates. Arch Gen Psychiatry 1985;42:225–32.

[5] Simon GE, VonKorff M. Prevalence, burden, and treatment of insomnia in primary care. Am J Psychiatry 1997;154:1417–23.

[6] Doi Y, Minowa M, Uchiyama M, et al. Subjective sleep quality and sleep problems in the general Japanese adult population. Psychiatry Clin Neurosci 2001;55:213–5.

[7] Fortner BV, Stepanski EJ, Wang SC, et al. Sleep and quality of life in breast cancer patients. J Pain Symptom Manage 2002;24:471–80.

[8] Rothenberg S, Zozula R, Funesti J, et al. Sleep habits in asymptomatic HIV-seropositive individuals. Sleep Research 1990;19:342.

[9] Cohen FL, Ferrans CE, Vizgirda V, et al. Sleep in men and women infected with human immunodeficiency virus. Holist Nurs Pract 1996;10: 33–43.

[10] Nokes KM, Kendrew J. Correlates of sleep quality in persons with HIV disease. J Assoc Nurses AIDS Care 2001;12:17–22.

[11] Rubinstein ML, Selwyn PA. High prevalence of insomnia in an outpatient population with HIV infection. Journal of Acquired Immune Deficiency Syndrome and Human Retrovirology 1998;19: 260–5.

[12] Üstün TB, Privett M, Lecrubier Y, et al. Form, frequency and burden of sleep problems in general health care: a report from the WHO Collaborative Study on Psychological Problems in General Health Care. Eur Psychiatry 1996;11: 5S–10S.

[13] Williams AB. Adherence to highly active antiretroviral therapy. Nurs Clin North Am 1999;34: 113–29.

[14] Simon V, Ho DD, Karim QA. HIV/AIDS epidemiology, pathogenesis, prevention, and treatment. Lancet 2006;368:489–504.

[15] UNAIDS. 2006 report on the global AIDS epidemic: a UNAIDS 10th anniversary special edition. Geneva: UNAIDS; 2006.

[16] Centers for Disease Control and Prevention. Epidemiology of HIV/AIDS—United States, 1981-2005. MMWR 2006;55:589–92.

[17] Staprans SI, Feinberg MB. Natural history and immunopathogenesis of HIV-1 disease. In: Sande MA, Volberding PA, editors. The medical management of AIDS. Philadelphia: W.B. Saunders; 1997. p. 29–56.

[18] Palella FJ, Delaney KM, Moorman AC, et al. Declining morbidity and mortality among patients with advanced human immunodeficiency virus infection. HIV Outpatient Study Investigators. N Engl J Med 1998;338:853–60.

[19] Walensky RP, Paltiel AD, Losina E, et al. The survival benefits of AIDS treatment in the United States. J Infect Dis 2006;194:11–9.

[20] Friedland GH, Williams A. Attaining higher goals in HIV treatment: the central importance of adherence. AIDS 1999;13:S61–72.

[21] Garcia de Olalla P, Knobel H, Carmona A, et al. Impact of adherence and highly active antiretroviral therapy on survival in HIV-infected patients. J Acquir Immune Defic Syndr 2002;30: 105–10.

[22] Darko DF, Mitler MM, Henriksen SJ. Lentiviral infection, immune response peptides and sleep. Adv Neuroimmunol 1995;5:57–77.

[23] Norman S, Shaukat M, Nay KN, et al. Alterations in sleep architecture in asymptomatic HIV seropositive patients. Sleep Research 1987;16:494.

[24] Norman SE, Chediak AD, Kiel M, et al. Sleep disturbances in HIV-infected homosexual men. AIDS 1990;4:775–81.

[25] White JL, Darko DF, Brown SJ, et al. Early central nervous system response to HIV infection: sleep distortion and cognitive-motor decrements. AIDS 1995;9:1043–50.

[26] Norman SE, Chediak A, Kiel M, et al. HIV infection and sleep: follow-up studies. Sleep Research 1990;19:339.

[27] Bell JE. An update on the neuropathology of HIV in the HAART era. Histopathology 2004;45: 549–59.

[28] Savard J, Morin CM. Insomnia in the context of cancer: a review of a neglected problem. J Clin Oncol 2001;19:895–908.

[29] Wiegand M, Möller AA, Schreiber W, et al. Nocturnal sleep EEG in patients with HIV infection. Eur Arch Psychiatry Clin Neurosci 1991;240: 153–8.

[30] Norman SE, Chediak AD, Freeman C, et al. Sleep disturbances in men with asymptomatic human immunodeficiency (HIV) infection. Sleep 1992; 15:150–5.

[31] Ferini-Strambi L, Oldani A, Tirloni G, et al. Slow wave sleep and cyclic alternating pattern (CAP) in HIV-infected asymptomatic men. Sleep 1995; 18:446–50.

[32] Brown S, Mitler M, Atkinson H, et al. Correlation of subjective sleep complaints, absolute T-4 cell number and anxiety in HIV illness. Sleep Research 1991;20:363.

[33] Wheatley D, Smith K. Clinical sleep patterns in human immune virus infection. Hum Psychopharmacol 1994;9:111–5.

[34] Perkins DO, Leserman J, Stern RA, et al. Somatic symptoms and HIV infection: relationship to depressive symptoms and indicators of HIV disease. Am J Psychiatry 1995;152:1776–81.

[35] Lee KA, Portillo CJ, Miramontes H. The influence of sleep and activity patterns on fatigue in women with HIV/AIDS. J Assoc Nurses AIDS Care 2001; 12(Suppl):19–27.

[36] Moeller AA, Oechsner M, Backmund HC, et al. Self-reported sleep quality in HIV infection: correlation to the stage of infection and zidovudine therapy. J Acquir Immune Defic Syndr 1991;4: 1000–3.

[37] Darko DF, McCutchan JA, Kripke DF, et al. Fatigue, sleep disturbance, disability, and indices of progression of HIV infection. Am J Psychiatry 1992;149:514–20.

[38] Kubicki S, Henkes H, Terstegge K, et al. AIDS-related sleep disturbances—a preliminary report. In: Kubicki, Henkes, Bienzle, Pohle, editors. HIV and the nervous system. Stuttgart (Germany): Gustav Fischer; 1988. p. 97–105.

[39] Terstegge K, Henkes H, Scheuler W, et al. Spectral power and coherence analysis of sleep EEG in AIDS patients: decrease in interhemispheric coherence. Sleep 1993;16:137–45.

[40] Richman DD, Fischl MA, Grieco MH, et al. The toxicity of azidothymine (AZT) in the treatment of patients with AIDS and AIDS-related complex: a double-blind, placebo-controlled trial. N Engl J Med 1987;317:192–7.

[41] Wichers M, van der Ven A, Maes M. Central nervous system symptoms related to the use of efavirenz in HIV-seropositive patients. Curr Opin Psychiatry 2002;15:643–7.

[42] Staszewski S, Morales-Ramirez J, Tashima KT, et al. Efavirenz plus zidovudine and lamivudine, efavirenz plus indinavir, and indinavir plus zidovudine and lamivudine in the treatment of HIV-1 infection in adults. Study 006 Team. N Engl J Med 1999;341:1865–73.

[43] de la Garza CL, Paoletti-Duarte S, Garcia-Martin C, et al. Efavirenz-induced psychosis. AIDS 2001;15:1911–2.

[44] Foster R, Olajide D, Everall I. Antiretroviral therapy-induced psychosis: case report and brief review of the literature. HIV Med 2003;4:139–44.

[45] Nuñez M, de Requena DG, Gallego L, et al. Higher efavirenz plasma levels correlate with development of insomnia. Journal of Acquired Immune Deficiency Syndrome and Human Retrovirology 2001;28:399.

[46] Fumaz CR, Tuldra A, Ferrer MJ, et al. Quality of life, emotional status, and adherence of HIV-1-infected patients treated with efavirenz versus protease inhibitor-containing regimens. Journal of Acquired Immune Deficiency Syndrome and Human Retrovirology 2002;29:244–53.

[47] Morlese JF, Qazi NA, Gazzard BG, et al. Nevirapine-induced neuropsychiatric complications, a class effect of non-nucleoside reverse transcriptase inhibitors? AIDS 2002;16:1840–1.

[48] Wise ME, Mistry K, Reid S. Neuropsychiatric complications of nevirapine treatment. BMJ 2002; 324:879.

[49] Holstein A, Plaschke A, Egberts E-H. Lipodystrophy and metabolic disorders as complication of antiretroviral therapy of HIV infection. Exp Clin Endocrinol Diabetes 2001;109:389–92.

[50] Martinez E, Mocroft A, Garcia-Viejo MA, et al. Risk of lipodystrophy in HIV-1-infected patients treated with protease inhibitors: a prospective cohort study. Lancet 2001;357:592–8.

[51] Lo Re V 3rd, Schutte-Rodin S, Kostman JR. Obstructive sleep apnoea among HIV patients. Int J STD AIDS 2006;17:614–20.

[52] Ford D, Kamerow D. Epidemiologic study of sleep disturbances and psychiatric disorders. JAMA 1989;262:1479–84.

[53] Henderson M, Safa F, Easterbrook P, et al. Fatigue among HIV-infected patients in the era of highly active antiretroviral therapy. HIV Med 2005;6: 347–52.

[54] Bing EG, Burnam MA, Longshore D, et al. Psychiatric disorders and drug use among human immunodeficiency virus-infected adults in the United States. Arch Gen Psychiatry 2001;58:721–8.

[55] Breitbart W. Pharmacotherapy of pain in AIDS. In: Wormser G, editor. A clinical guide to AIDS and HIV. Philadelphia: Lippincott-Raven; 1996. p. 359–78.

[56] Sutton DA, Moldofsky H, Badley EM. Insomnia and health problems in Canadians. Sleep 2001; 24:665–70.

[57] Singer EJ, Zorilla C, Fahy-Chandon B, et al. Painful symptoms reported by ambulatory HIV-infected men in a longitudinal study. Pain 1993;54:15–9.

[58] Larue F, Fontaine A, Colleau SM. Underestimation and undertreatment of pain in HIV disease: multicentre study. BMJ 1997;314:23–23.

[59] American Sleep Disorders Association. The international classification of sleep disorders: diagnostic and coding nanual. Rochester (MN): American Sleep Disorders Association; 1997.

[60] Kupfer DJ, Reynolds CF III. Management of insomnia. N Engl J Med 1997;336:341–6.

[61] Dreher HM. The effect of caffeine reduction on sleep quality and well-being in persons with HIV. J Psychosom Res 2003;54:191–8.

[62] Nowell PD, Mazumdar S, Buysse DJ, et al. Benzo-diazepines an zolpidem for chronic insomnia: a meta-analysis of treatment efficacy. JAMA 1997; 278:2170–7.

[63] Holbrook AM, Crowther R, Lotter A, et al. Meta-analysis of benzodiazepine use in the treatment of insomnia. Can Med Assoc J 2000;162: 225–33.

[64] Smith MT, Perlis ML, Park A, et al. Comparative meta-analysis of pharmacotherapy and behavior therapy for persistent insomnia. Am J Psychiatry 2002;159:5–11.

[65] Morin CM, Culbert JP, Schwartz SM. Nonphar-macological interventions for insomnia: a meta-analysis of treatment efficacy. Am J Psychiatry 1994;151:1172–80.

[66] Murtagh DRR, Greenwood KM. Identifying effective psychological treatments for insomnia: a meta-analysis. J Consult Clin Psychol 1995;63: 79–89.

SLEEP
MEDICINE
CLINICS

Sleep Med Clin 2 (2007) 59–66

Sleep Disorders and End-Stage Renal Disease

Patrick Hanly, MD, FRCPC, D ABSM

- Insomnia
- Daytime sleepiness
- Restless legs syndrome and periodic limb movement disorder
  Prevalence and presentation
  Clinical significance
  Pathogenesis
  Treatment
- Sleep apnea
  Prevalence
  Presentation
  Clinical significance
  Pathogenesis
  Treatment
- Acknowledgments
- References

Sleep complaints and sleep disorders are common in patients with end-stage renal disease (ESRD). Patients frequently report both insomnia and excessive sleepiness, which are significant contributors to their impaired quality of life. Restless legs syndrome, periodic limb movement disorder, and sleep apnea are highly prevalent. In addition to causing sleep disruption and sleep loss, these conditions may further increase the considerable cardiovascular morbidity and mortality in this patient population. Although conventional dialysis does not correct these sleep disorders, nocturnal hemodialysis and renal transplantation may be more effective.

Insomnia

Insomnia is a common complaint in patients with end-stage renal disease (ESRD) and the prevalence appears to be similar regardless of the mode of dialysis. In one study, insomnia was reported by 52% of patients on chronic hemodialysis, 50% of patients on chronic ambulatory peritoneal dialysis, and 12% of a matched healthy control group [1]. Similar findings have been reported in other studies of subjective sleep complaints in this patient population [2–8]. The etiology is multifactorial and includes sleep disruption associated with restless legs syndrome, periodic limb movement disorder, and sleep apnea, metabolic factors such as uremia, anemia, hypercalcemia, bone pain and pruritus, psychiatric disorders such as depression, circadian rhythm disorders such as delayed sleep phase syndrome [2], medications, and poor sleep hygiene including frequent napping during daytime dialysis. Patients report that insomnia is a significant source of stress, which impairs their quality of life [9,10].

In addition to subjective sleep complaints, there is objective evidence of both sleep loss and sleep disruption in patients with ESRD. Polysomnographic studies have reported a total sleep time of 4.4 to 6 hours, fragmented by a high frequency of arousals (up to 30 per hour), resulting in a sleep efficiency that ranged from 66% to 85% [11–16]. Sleep architecture varies between studies but, generally, stage 1 and 2 non-rapid eye movement (NREM) sleep is increased whereas slow wave sleep and REM sleep are reduced [11,14,15,17,18].

Sleep Centre, Foothills Medical Centre, 1421 Health Sciences Centre, 3330 Hospital Drive NW, Calgary, Alberta, T2N 4N1 Canada
E-mail address: phanly@ucalgary.ca

Daytime sleepiness

The prevalence of *subjective* daytime sleepiness, assessed by a standardized questionnaire, has been reported in 52% to 67% of patients on chronic dialysis [2,18]. *Objective* daytime sleepiness can be evaluated by the multiple sleep latency test (MSLT) [19], which has been used in three studies in this patient population.

Stepanski and colleagues [18] evaluated 18 patients who reported insomnia and/or daytime sleepiness. Eleven (61%) patients had sleep apnea. The mean sleep latency was 6.6 ± 3.7 minutes and it was significantly lower in those with apnea (5.5 ± 4.0 minutes) than those without apnea (7.7 ± 2.9 minutes). This study is limited by the small sample size and selection of patients with sleep complaints who may not be representative of the general ESRD population.

Hanly and colleagues [12] evaluated 24 patients on conventional hemodialysis (CHD). There was no prior assessment of sleep symptoms and, consequently, patients were not selected on the basis of an underlying sleep disorder. Daytime sleepiness was assessed subjectively by the Epworth Sleepiness Scale (ESS) [20] and objectively by the MSLT. Subjective sleepiness (ESS < 8) was reported in 50% of patients and objective sleepiness (sleep latency < 5 minutes) was found in 50% of patients. However, there was no correlation between the ESS scores and the MSLT results indicating that the patients who reported sleepiness were not objectively sleepy and vice versa.

To identify potential determinants of daytime sleepiness, patients were divided into somnolent and alert groups based on a sleep latency of 5 minutes. There were no significant intergroup differences in the prevalence of coexisting medical disorders, hemoglobin, sedating medications, gender, age, body mass index, sleep architecture, apnea-hypopnea index (AHI), or nocturnal oxygen saturation. However, somnolent patients were significantly more uremic and had more periodic limb movements (PLM). In addition, a significant correlation was found between the BUN (blood urea nitrogen) and mean sleep latency (r = −0.58, P = .008). Fifteen of these patients were converted to nocturnal hemodialysis (NHD). In the somnolent group, there was a trend for the frequency of periodic limb movements to fall and a corresponding trend for sleep latency to increase, whereas in the alert group there was a trend for the frequency of PLM to increase and a corresponding trend for sleep latency to fall. When the data from these 2 groups were combined, a significant correlation was found between the *change* in PLM and the *change* in sleep latency (r = −0.63, P = .021)

(Fig. 1). These results indicate that daytime sleepiness is common in unselected patients with ESRD and that it is correlated with the level of uremia and the presence of periodic limb movements. Taken at face value, these data suggest a potential role for the treatment of PLM in this population.

Finally, Parker and colleagues [16] evaluated 46 patients on CHD following exclusion of those with known causes of daytime sleepiness such as chronic medical disorders associated with sleep disruption, central nervous system (CNS) medications, and a history suggestive of sleep disorders such as sleep apnea, restless legs syndrome, or periodic limb movement disorder (PLMD). Despite this screening, 50% of patients had sleep apnea and 50% had PLMD. Thirteen percent of patients had evidence of "pathological" sleepiness reflected by sleep latency less than 5 minutes and a further 33% had mild daytime sleepiness (sleep latency 5 to 10 minutes). In addition, 48% of patients had REM sleep on at least one nap, and 17% of patients had REM sleep on two or more naps.

These findings further support the high prevalence of daytime sleepiness in patients with ESRD. Although mild sleep apnea was present in some patients, the respiratory disturbance index (RDI) accounted for only 11% of the variance in the measures of sleepiness, which implies that nonrespiratory factors play a significant role. The high prevalence of REM sleep during daytime naps may simply reflect the severity of nighttime sleep disruption or, alternatively, may indicate a basic

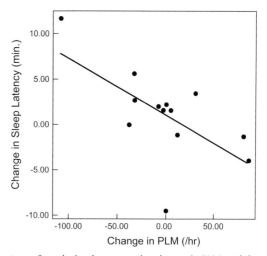

Fig. 1. Correlation between the *change* in PLM and the *change* in sleep latency (MSLT) after conversion from conventional hemodialysis to nocturnal hemodialysis (R = −0.63; P = .021). Paired data points available for 13 patients. (*From* Hanly PJ, Gabor JY, Chan C, et al. Daytime sleepiness in patients with CRF: impact of nocturnal hemodialysis. Am J Kidney Dis 2003;41: 403–10; with permission.)

desynchronization of the timing of REM sleep. The investigators offered several potential explanations for the pathogenesis of daytime sleepiness in this patient population, including subclinical uremic encephalopathy [21], deficiency of tyrosine [22], which is an important precursor in the metabolism of dopamine, release of sleep-inducing inflammatory cytokines during dialysis [23], persistence of melatonin during the daytime [24], and alteration of body temperature rhythm, which is closely associated with the sleep-wakefulness rhythm [25].

Restless legs syndrome and periodic limb movement disorder

Prevalence and presentation

Restless legs syndrome (RLS) and PLMD have characteristic clinical and polysomnographic features, which have been well described [26]. RLS has been reported in up to 80% of patients with ESRD [2,3,27,28], which is remarkably higher than the prevalence in the general population (5% to 15%) [26]. Although the reported prevalence of PLMD in patients with ESRD has varied considerably, it is generally higher than 50% [2,3,26,27,29–32].

Clinical significance

The restlessness experienced by patients with RLS may be problematic both during the daytime, especially during inactivity, and at nighttime when patients report difficulty initiating and maintaining sleep [2,30]. It is more challenging to determine whether PLMD is responsible for complaints of sleep disruption, and in some patients a trial of pharmacologic therapy may be required to resolve this. A less apparent potential clinical consequence of RLS and PLMD is the interesting association that has been reported between them and increased mortality in patients with ESRD [28,33] Although the underlying mechanism for such an association has not been determined, potential explanations include poor compliance with therapy and the hemodynamic consequences of recurrent sleep disruption [34].

Pathogenesis

The pathophysiology of RLS and PLM in patients with ESRD is not understood. However, common risk factors in this patient population that are recognized to exacerbate, if not cause, these sleep disorders include anemia, iron deficiency, and peripheral and CNS abnormalities [26,35]. In addition, it is likely that alteration of dopamine and opioid activity in the nervous system plays a role. Correction of anemia by treatment with erythropoietin was associated with reduction in the frequency of PLMD, improvement in sleep quality, and daytime alertness [36]. Iron deficiency has the potential to play a dual role in that it can cause anemia and is also a cofactor in the metabolism of dopamine in the brain. Accordingly, treatment with intravenous iron was associated with a significant improvement in RLS and PLM [37] Peripheral neuropathy, secondary to uremia or the underlying cause of ESRD (such as diabetes) may also predispose patients to develop RLS and/or PLMD.

Treatment

The management of RLS and PLMD consists of general measures, specific pharmacologic therapy, and renal function replacement. General measures include reduction of potential exacerbating factors such as lifestyle factors (excess caffeine, alcohol, and nicotine), medical conditions (anemia, iron deficiency), and medications (tricyclic antidepressants, serotonin re-uptake inhibitors, dopamine antagonists). Medications used to treat RLS and PLMD include L-dopa [38–40] and dopamine agonists such as pergolide [41], pramipexole [42], and ropinirole [43]. These are favored over benzodiazepines such as clonazepam [44] and opiates, which may not be as effective and are more likely to be associated with drowsiness and dependence. Although neither conventional hemodialysis, peritoneal dialysis, or nocturnal hemodialysis have been shown to correct RLS or PLMD, renal transplantation has been associated with an improvement in RLS [45,46].

Sleep apnea

Prevalence

A variety of studies have reported that more than 50% of ESRD patients have sleep apnea [13,17,18,47–50], which is dramatically higher than the prevalence in the general population (2% to 4%) [51]. Although some of these studies may be limited by selection bias and others were not controlled for the influence of comorbid disease, there is little doubt that sleep apnea is common in patients with ESRD. In addition, the prevalence appears to be similar in predialysis patients and those treated with peritoneal dialysis or hemodialysis [17,50], which suggests that the pathophysiology of sleep apnea in this population is linked to ESRD itself rather than the initiation or mode of dialysis.

Presentation

The clinical presentation of sleep apnea in patients with ESRD is similar to that in patients with normal renal function in that bed-partners may witness apneas during sleep and patients experience daytime sleepiness [52,53] but differs in that snoring is reported to be less intense [54] and patients are generally lighter in weight [18]. However, some of the characteristic symptoms of sleep apnea such as fatigue, depression, and impaired cognitive and sexual function [52] may be mistakenly attributed to chronic renal failure (CRF) itself [47,49] or to comorbid conditions, which has probably resulted in the underrecognition of sleep apnea in this population over the years.

Clinical significance

The coexistence of untreated sleep apnea in a large proportion of patients with ESRD has many potential clinical consequences. First, sleep apnea may exacerbate the symptoms of CRF, such as daytime fatigue, sleepiness, and impaired neurocognitive function [55], which may hinder renal rehabilitation. Second, sleep apnea may exacerbate the cardiovascular complications of ESRD, which are the leading causes of morbidity and mortality in these patients [56]. The annual mortality rate of patients with ESRD is more than 20% [33]. Sleep apnea independently increases the prevalence of systemic hypertension [57–59], coronary artery disease [60–62], and cerebrovascular disease [63,64] and also exacerbates myocardial ischemia in patients with coexisting coronary artery disease [65,66]. More recently, sleep apnea has been identified as a source of increased oxidative stress [67] and systemic inflammation [68], which may accelerate the development of atherosclerosis [69]. Third, sleep apnea may exacerbate the infectious complications common in ESRD patients, because sleep disruption and sleep deprivation degrade immune function [70]. Finally, coexisting sleep apnea may increase the risk of death in this patient population [71]. Consequently, there is great potential for the diagnosis and treatment of sleep apnea to improve both the quality of life and survival in CRF patients.

Pathogenesis

The pathogenesis of sleep apnea in ESRD is not clear, although many hypotheses have been considered [48–50,72]. Several investigators have observed features of both obstructive and central sleep apnea [11,13,72–74], which supports the hypothesis that the pathogenesis of sleep apnea in patients with CRF is attributable to both destabilization of central ventilatory control and upper airway occlusion.

A recent study by Beecroft and colleagues [75] demonstrated enhanced ventilatory sensitivity to hypercapnia in ESRD patients, which was positively correlated with apnea severity. This destabilizes respiratory control by increasing feedback and therefore "loop gain" [76]. Although altered chemoreflex responsiveness has been well described in the pathogenesis of central sleep apnea [77–79], most patients in this study had obstructive sleep apnea However, there is abundant evidence that oscillation in respiratory control does occur in patients with obstructive sleep apnea (OSA). Periodic breathing was observed over 20 years ago following tracheostomy for the treatment of severe OSA [80,81] and more recently, ventilatory instability, reflected by a high loop gain, has been reported in patients with severe OSA [82]. Although this cross-sectional study established a significant association between ventilatory instability and sleep apnea in patients with ESRD, further studies are required to establish causality between these two phenomena.

Alternatively, patients with ESRD may develop sleep apnea through mechanisms that promote upper airway occlusion during sleep. Such patients are vulnerable to fluid overload by virtue of their oliguria and intermittent dialysis. Hypervolemia is common in patients with ESRD and could contribute to pharyngeal narrowing if it were localized to the upper airway. Although interstitial edema has been observed in upper airway tissue in OSA patients with normal renal function [83], whether these changes contribute to pharyngeal narrowing has not been fully explored. Hypervolemia may also lead to pharyngeal narrowing through increasing fluid volume in the neck and peripharyngeal structures. Impedance of venous return to the heart through cuff inflation on the legs has been shown to increase cross-sectional area of the upper airway [84], whereas displacement of fluid from the lower limbs has recently been reported to increase neck circumference and pharyngeal resistance [85]. Another potential cause of pharyngeal narrowing is upper airway dilator muscle dysfunction as a result of neuropathy or myopathy associated with chronic uremia or the underlying cause of ESRD, such as diabetes mellitus [13]. Both sensory neuropathy [86] and muscle denervation [87] have been demonstrated in the upper airway in OSA patients with normal renal function and may play a role in exacerbating the disease process in patients with ESRD.

Finally, the potential role of oxidative stress, inflammatory cytokines, and middle molecules, all of which are elevated in ESRD, in the development of ventilatory instability and/or upper airway occlusion needs to be addressed.

Treatment

Conventional management of sleep apnea includes treatment of underlying medical conditions such as obesity or hypothyroidism, correction of potential aggravating factors such as sleeping in the supine position, taking alcohol or sedatives close to bedtime, and mechanical devices such as a dental appliance or continuous positive airway pressure (CPAP) to keep the upper airway open during sleep. There has been surprisingly little investigation of these commonly used therapies in patients with ESRD. A single study in a small group of patients treated with CPAP reported a similar compliance rate as that seen in patients with normal renal function [74]. However, this may not be a consistent finding; anecdotal clinical experience indicates that the multifactorial etiology of sleep disruption in ESRD patients makes it more difficult to tolerate CPAP therapy. The role of upper airway surgery has not been specifically addressed in patients with ESRD but it is not likely to be better than in patients with normal renal function. Supplemental oxygen may be useful in patients who have a significant amount of central apnea, particularly Cheyne-Stokes respiration associated with heart failure [88], but this has not been evaluated.

Sleep apnea is not corrected by conventional hemodialysis or peritoneal dialysis [13,17,50]. Apnea frequency has been reduced by the use of bicarbonate rather than an acetate-based dialysate [89]. There is a single case report of resolution of sleep apnea in a critically ill patient who received intensive daily hemodialysis [90]. Nocturnal hemodialysis (NHD), which enables patients to receive hemodialysis at home during sleep, six nights per week for 6 to 8 hours per night, has been shown to improve sleep apnea [11]. Following conversion from CHD to NHD, there was a significant reduction in AHI from 25 ± 25 per hour to 8 ± 8 per hour. These changes were more dramatic in the seven subjects who had significant sleep apnea in whom the AHI fell from 46 ± 19 per hour on CHD to 9 ± 9 per hour (Fig. 2). Although case reports have indicated correction of sleep apnea following successful kidney transplantation [72,91], preliminary results from a case series suggest that sleep apnea resolves in only a minority of patients following transplantation [92]. The persistence of sleep apnea following kidney transplantation may be related to nonrenal factors such as weight gain and a medication effect on the upper airway and requires further study.

Acknowledgments

The author is grateful to Ms Patty Nielsen for her clerical assistance.

References

[1] Holley JL, Nespor S, Rault R. Characterizing sleep disorders in chronic hemodialysis patients. ASAIO Trans 1991;37:M456–7.

[2] Walker S, Fine A, Kryger MH. Sleep complaints are common in a dialysis unit. Am J Kidney Dis 1995;26:751–6.

[3] Hui DS, Wong TY, Ko FW, et al. Prevalence of sleep disturbances in Chinese patients with end-stage renal failure on continuous ambulatory peritoneal dialysis. Am J Kidney Dis 2000; 36:783–8.

[4] Venmans BJ, van Kralingen KW, Chandi DD, et al. Sleep complaints and sleep disordered breathing in hemodialysis patients. Neth J Med 1999;54:207–12.

[5] Burmann-Urbanek M, Sanner B, Laschewski F, et al. [Sleep disorders in patients with dialysis-dependent renal failure]. Pneumologie 1995; 49(Suppl 1):158–60.

[6] Yoshioka M, Ishii T, Fukunishi I. Sleep disturbance of end-stage renal disease. Jpn J Psychiatry Neurol 1993;47:847–51.

[7] Abella, Rodriguez M, Merino D, Grizzo M, et al. Sleep disorders in hemodialysis patients. Transplant Proc 1999;31:3082.

[8] Unruh ML, Hartunian MG, Chapman MM, et al. Sleep quality and clinical correlates in patients on maintenance dialysis. Clin Nephrol 2003; 59:280–8.

[9] Molzahn AE, Northcott HC, Dossetor JB. Quality of life of individuals with end stage renal disease: perceptions of patients, nurses, and physicians. ANNA J 1997;24:325–33.

[10] Parfrey PS, Vavasour HM, Henry S, et al. Clinical features and severity of nonspecific symptoms in dialysis patients. Nephron 1988;50:121–8.

[11] Hanly PJ, Pierratos A. Improvement of sleep apnea in patients with chronic renal failure who undergo nocturnal hemodialysis. N Engl J Med 2001;344(2):102–7.

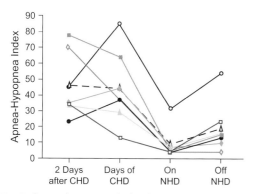

Fig. 2. Apnea-hypopnea index in seven patients with a baseline apnea-hypopnea index higher than 15. CHD denotes conventional hemodialysis, and NHD nocturnal hemodialysis. The mean values are represented by the broken black line. (*From* Hanly PJ, Pierratos A. Improvement of sleep apnea in patients with chronic renal failure who undergo nocturnal hemodialysis. N Engl J Med 2001;344(2):102–7.)

[12] Hanly PJ, Gabor JY, Chan C, et al. Daytime sleepiness in patients with CRF: impact of nocturnal hemodialysis. Am J Kidney Dis 2003;41:403–10.

[13] Mendelson WB, Wadhwa NK, Greenberg HE, et al. Effects of hemodialysis on sleep apnea syndrome in end-stage renal disease. Clin Nephrol 1990;33:247–51.

[14] Wadhwa NK, Seliger M, Greenberg HE, et al. Sleep-related respiratory disorders in end-stage renal disease patients on peritoneal dialysis. Perit Dial Int 1992;12:51–6.

[15] Hallett MD, Burden S, Stewart D, et al. Sleep apnea in ESRD patients on HD and CAPD. Perit Dial Int 1996;16(Suppl 1):S429–33.

[16] Parker KP, Bliwise DL, Bailey JL, et al. Daytime sleepiness in stable hemodialysis patients. Am J Kidney Dis 2003;41:394–402.

[17] Wadhwa NK, Mendelson WB. A comparison of sleep-disordered respiration in ESRD patients receiving hemodialysis and peritoneal dialysis. Adv Perit Dial 1992;8:195–8.

[18] Stepanski E, Faber M, Zorick F, et al. Sleep disorders in patients on continuous ambulatory peritoneal dialysis. J Am Soc Nephrol 1995;6:192–7.

[19] Carskadon MA, Dement WC, Mitler MM, et al. Guidelines for the multiple sleep latency test (MSLT): a standard measure of sleepiness. Sleep 1986;9:519–24.

[20] Johns JW. A new method for measuring daytime sleepiness: the Epworth sleepiness scale. Sleep 1991;14:540–5.

[21] Hughes JR. Correlations between EEG and chemical changes in uremia. Electroencephalogr Clin Neurophysiol 1980;48:583–94.

[22] Furst P. Amino acid metabolism in uremia. J Am Coll Nutr 1989;8:310–23.

[23] Rousseau Y, Haeffner-Cavaillon N, Poignet JL, et al. In vivo intracellular cytokine production by leukocytes during haemodialysis. Cytokine 2000;12:506–17.

[24] Vaziri ND, Oveisi F, Wierszbiezki M, et al. Serum melatonin and 6-sulfatoxymelatonin in end-stage renal disease: effect of hemodialysis. Artif Organs 1993;17:764–9.

[25] Parker KP, Bliwise DL, Rye DB. Hemodialysis disrupts basic sleep regulatory mechanisms: building hypotheses. Nurs Res 2000;49:327–32.

[26] Sateia MJ, editor. The international classification of sleep disorders. 2nd edition (Diagnostic and coding manual). Westchester (PA): American Academy of Sleep Medicine; 2005. p. 178–82.

[27] Holley JL, Nespor S, Rault R. A comparison of reported sleep disorders in patients on chronic hemodialysis and continuous peritoneal dialysis. Am J Kidney Dis 1992;19:156–61.

[28] Unruh ML, Levey AS, D'Ambrosio C, et al. Restless legs symptoms among incident dialysis patients: association with lower quality of life and shorter survival. Am J Kidney Dis 2004;43:900–9.

[29] Takaki J, Nishi T, Nangaku M, et al. Clinical and psychological aspects of restless legs syndrome in uremic patients on hemodialysis. Am J Kidney Dis 2003;41:833–9.

[30] Winkelman JW, Chertow GM, Lazarus JM. Restless legs syndrome in end-stage renal disease. Am J Kidney Dis 1996;28:372–8.

[31] Huiqi Q, Shan L, Mingcai Q. Restless legs syndrome (RLS) in uremic patients is related to the frequency of hemodialysis sessions. Nephron 2000;86:540.

[32] Miranda M, Araya F, Castillo JL, et al. Restless legs syndrome: a clinical study in adult general population and in uremic patients. Rev Med Chil 2001;129:179–86.

[33] Benz RL, Pressman MR, Hovick ET, et al. Potential novel predictors of mortality in end-stage renal disease patients with sleep disorders. Am J Kidney Dis 2000;35:1052–60.

[34] Ali NJ, Davies RJ, Fleetham JA, et al. Periodic movements of the legs during sleep associated with rises in systemic blood pressure. Sleep 1991;14:163–5.

[35] Gigli GL, Adorati M, Dolso P, et al. Restless legs syndrome in end-stage renal disease. Sleep Med 2004;5:309–15.

[36] Benz RL, Pressman MR, Hovick ET, et al. A preliminary study of the effects of correction of anemia with recombinant human erythropoietin therapy on sleep, sleep disorders, and daytime sleepiness in hemodialysis patients (The SLEEPO study). Am J Kidney Dis 1999;34:1089–95.

[37] Sloand JA, Shelly MA, Feigin A, et al. A double-blind, placebo-controlled trial of intravenous iron dextran therapy in patients with ESRD and restless legs syndrome. Am J Kidney Dis 2004;43:663–70.

[38] Walker SL, Fine A, Kryger MH. L-DOPA/carbidopa for nocturnal movement disorders in uremia. Sleep 1996;19:214–8.

[39] Sandyk R, Bernick C, Lee SM, et al. L-dopa in uremic patients with the restless legs syndrome. Int J Neurosci 1987;35:233–5.

[40] Trenkwalder C, Stiasny K, Pollmacher T, et al. L-dopa therapy of uremic and idiopathic restless legs syndrome: a double-blind, crossover trial. Sleep 1995;18:681–8.

[41] Pieta J, Millar T, Zacharias J, et al. Effect of pergolide on restless legs and leg movements in sleep in uremic patients. Sleep 1998;21:617–22.

[42] Miranda M, Kagi M, Fabres L, et al. Pramipexole for the treatment of uremic restless legs in patients undergoing hemodialysis. Neurology 2004;62:831–2.

[43] Pellecchia MT, Vitale C, Sabatini M, et al. Ropinirole as a treatment of restless legs syndrome in patients on chronic hemodialysis: an open randomized crossover trial versus levodopa sustained release. Clin Neuropharmacol 2004;27:178–81.

[44] Braude W, Barnes T. Clonazepam: effective treatment for restless legs syndrome in uraemia. Br Med J (Clin Res Ed) 1982;284:510.

[45] Molnar MZ, Novak M, Ambrus C, et al. Restless legs syndrome in patients after renal transplantation. Am J Kidney Dis 2005;45:388–96.

[46] Winkelmann J, Stautner A, Samtleben W, et al. Long-term course of restless legs syndrome in dialysis patients after kidney transplantation. Mov Disord 2002;17:1072–6.

[47] Kimmel PL. Sleep disorders in chronic renal disease. J Nephrol 1989;1:59–65.

[48] Fletcher EC. Obstructive sleep apnea and the kidney. J Am Soc Nephrol 1993;4:1111–21.

[49] Kraus MA, Hamburger RJ. Sleep apnea in renal failure. Adv Perit Dial 1997;13:88–92.

[50] Kimmel PL, Miller G, Mendelson WB. Sleep apnea syndrome in chronic renal disease. Am J Med 1989;86:308–14.

[51] Young T, Palta M, Dempsey J, et al. The occurrence of sleep-disordered breathing among middle-aged adults. N Engl J Med 1993;328:1230–5.

[52] Guilleminault C. Clinical features and evaluation of obstructive sleep apnea. In: Kryger M, Roth T, Dement WC, editors. Principles and practices of sleep medicine. 2nd edition. Philadelphia: W.B. Saunders; 1994. p. 667–77.

[53] Hanly P, Zuberi-Khokhar N. Daytime sleepiness in patients with congestive heart failure and Cheyne-Stokes respiration. Chest 1995;107: 952–8.

[54] Parker KP, Bliwise DL. Clinical comparison of hemodialysis and sleep apnea patients with excessive daytime sleepiness. ANNA J 1997;24: 663–5.

[55] Heslegrave R, Thornley K, Ouwendyk M, et al. Impact of nocturnal hemodialysis on sleep and daytime cognitive functioning in patients with chronic renal failure. Sleep 1998;21:51.

[56] Bloembergen WE, Port FK, Mauger EA, et al. A comparison of cause of death between patients treated with hemodialysis and peritoneal dialysis. J Am Soc Nephrol 1995;6:184–91.

[57] Hla KM, Young TB, Bidwell T, et al. Sleep apnea and hypertension. A population-based study. Ann Intern Med 1994;120:382–8.

[58] Peppard PE, Young T, Palta M, et al. Prospective study of the association between sleep-disordered breathing and hypertension. N Engl J Med 2000;342:1378–84.

[59] Lavie P, Herer P, Hoffstein V. Obstructive sleep apnoea syndrome as a risk factor for hypertension: population study. Br Med J 2000;320: 479–82.

[60] Hung J, Whitford EG, Parsons RW, et al. Association of sleep apnoea with myocardial infarction in men. Lancet 1990;336:261–4.

[61] Peker Y, Hedner J, Kraiczi H, et al. Respiratory disturbance index: an independent predictor of mortality in coronary artery disease. Am J Respir Crit Care Med 2000;162:81–6.

[62] Marin JM, Carrizo SJ, Vicente E, et al. Long-term cardiovascular outcomes in men with obstructive sleep apnoea-hypopnoea with or without treatment with continuous positive airway pressure: an observational study. Lancet 2005; 365:1046–53.

[63] Spriggs DA, French JM, Murdy JM, et al. Snoring increases the risk of stroke and adversely affects prognosis. Q J Med 1992;83:555–62.

[64] Yaggi HK, Concato J, Kernan WN, et al. Obstructive sleep apnea as a risk factor for stroke and death. N Engl J Med 2005;353:2034–41.

[65] Hanly P, Sasson Z, Zuberi N, et al. ST-segment depression during sleep in obstructive sleep apnea. Am J Cardiol 1993;71:1341–5.

[66] Mooe T, Franklin KA, Wiklund U, et al. Sleep disordered breathing and myocardial ischemia in patients with coronary artery disease. Chest 2000;117:1597–602.

[67] Lavie L. Obstructive sleep apnoea syndrome—an oxidative stress disorder. Sleep Med Rev 2003;7: 35–51.

[68] Larkin EK, Rosen CL, Kirchner HL, et al. Variation of C-reactive protein levels in adolescents: association with sleep-disordered breathing and sleep duration. Circulation 2005;111: 1978–84.

[69] Lavie L. Sleep-disordered breathing and cerebrovascular disease: a mechanistic approach. Neurol Clin 2005;23:1059–75.

[70] Benca RM, Quintas J. Sleep and host defenses: a review. Sleep 1997;20:1027–37.

[71] Charest AF, Hanly PJ, Parkes RK, et al. Impact of sleep apnea on mortality in patients with end-stage renal disease. J Am Soc Nephrol 2004;15: 637A.

[72] Langevin B, Fouque D, Leger P, et al. Sleep apnea syndrome and end-stage renal disease. Cure after renal transplantation. Chest 1993;103:1330–5.

[73] Onal E. Sleep-disordered breathing in patients with end-stage renal disease. Kidney 1993;2: 309–11.

[74] Pressman MR, Benz RL, Schleifer CR, et al. Sleep disordered breathing in ESRD: acute beneficial effects of treatment with nasal continuous positive airway pressure. Kidney Int 1993;43:1134–9.

[75] Beecroft J, Duffin J, Pierratos A, et al. Enhanced chemo-responsiveness in patients with sleep apnoea and end-stage renal disease. Eur Respir J 2006;28:151–8.

[76] Khoo MC. Determinants of ventilatory instability and variability. Respir Physiol 2000;122: 167–82.

[77] Xie A, Rutherford R, Rankin F, et al. Hypocapnia and increased ventilatory responsiveness in patients with idiopathic central sleep apnea. Am J Respir Crit Care Med 1995;152:1950–5.

[78] Lahiri S, Maret K, Sherpa MG. Dependence of high altitude sleep apnea on ventilatory sensitivity to hypoxia. Respir Physiol 1983;52:281–301.

[79] Javaheri S. A mechanism of central sleep apnea in patients with heart failure. N Engl J Med 1999;341:949–54.

[80] Onal E, Lopata M. Periodic breathing and the pathogenesis of occlusive sleep apneas. Am Rev Respir Dis 1982;126:676–80.

[81] Weitzman ED, Kahn E, Pollak CP. Quantitative analysis of sleep and sleep apnea before and after tracheostomy in patients with the hypersomnia-sleep apnea syndrome. Sleep 1980;3:407–23.

[82] Younes M, Ostrowski M, Thompson W, et al. Chemical control stability in patients with obstructive sleep apnea. Am J Respir Crit Care Med 2001;163:1181–90.

[83] Anastassov GE, Trieger N. Edema in the upper airway in patients with obstructive sleep apnea syndrome. Oral Surg Oral Med Oral Pathol Oral Radiol Endod 1998;86:644–7.

[84] Shepard JW Jr, Pevernagie DA, Stanson AW, et al. Effects of changes in central venous pressure on upper airway size in patients with obstructive sleep apnea. Am J Respir Crit Care Med 1996;153:250–4.

[85] Chiu KL, Ryan CM, Shiota S, et al. Fluid shift by lower body positive pressure increases pharyngeal resistance in healthy subjects. Am J Respir Crit Care Med 2006;174:1378–83.

[86] Kimoff RJ, Sforza E, Champagne V, et al. Upper airway sensation in snoring and obstructive sleep apnea. Am J Respir Crit Care Med 2001;164: 250–5.

[87] Boyd JH, Petrof BJ, Hamid Q, et al. Upper airway muscle inflammation and denervation changes in obstructive sleep apnea. Am J Respir Crit Care Med 2004;170:541–6.

[88] Hanly PJ, Millar TW, Steljes DG, et al. The effect of oxygen on respiration and sleep in patients with congestive heart failure. Ann Intern Med 1989;111:777–82.

[89] Jean G, Piperno D, Francois B, et al. Sleep apnea incidence in maintenance hemodialysis patients: influence of dialysate buffer. Nephron 1995;71: 138–42.

[90] Fein AM, Niederman MS, Imbriano L, et al. Reversal of sleep apnea in uremia by dialysis. Arch Intern Med 1987;147:1355–6.

[91] Auckley DH, Schmidt-Nowara W, Brown LK. Reversal of sleep apnea hypopnea syndrome in end-stage renal disease after kidney transplantation. Am J Kidney Dis 1999;34: 739–44.

[92] Beecroft J, Zaltzman J, Prasad R, et al. Evaluation of sleep apnea in patients with chronic renal failure treated with kidney transplantation. Proc Am Thorac Soc 2006;3:A568.

ELSEVIER
SAUNDERS

SLEEP
MEDICINE
CLINICS

Sleep Med Clin 2 (2007) 67–75

Sleep and Cancer

Edward J. Stepanski, PhD[a],*, Helen J. Burgess, PhD[b]

Sleep-related problems, such as insomnia, fatigue, and daytime sleepiness are extremely common in patients with cancer according to a number of studies describing patient-reported outcomes [1–3]. Research in this area has been largely descriptive, and there have been few systematic studies aimed at understanding the etiology or consequences of poor sleep in this patient population [4]. Research investigating quality of life (QoL) in cancer patients has found that poor sleep is an important predictor of decreased QoL [2,5]. There is a recent trend toward increased study of sleep of patients with cancer. A growing literature investigating links between sleep quantity and quality and immune system function and inflammation markers has relevance to patients receiving treatment for cancer [6–8]. Finally, there are provocative, but controversial, findings regarding integration of knowledge from biological rhythms research into clinical practice regarding the timing of delivery of chemotherapy.

Prevalence of sleep complaints in cancer

The prevalence of sleep complaints in patients with cancer varies dramatically among studies, but consistently higher rates of insomnia are reported in patients with cancer, compared with the general population or a control group [2,9–12]. These estimates may vary because of differences in the methodology used to assess sleep complaints, or because of differences in the sample characteristics of cancer patients for a given study. This variability is consistent with what is found for prevalence estimates for insomnia throughout the literature in noncancer populations [13].

The prevalence of insomnia was reported as 32% in a group 1012 patients heterogeneous with respect to type and stage of cancer [9], and was 63% in a sample of 97 women with metastatic breast cancer [10]. Those studies used short sleep questionnaires to assess for the presence of sleep complaints. Studies using a validated self-report measure, the

[a] Accelerated Community Oncology Research Network, 1770 Kirby Parkway, Suite 400, Memphis, TN 38138, USA
[b] Present address: Biological Rhythms Research Laboratory, Rush University Medical Center, 1645 West Jackson Blvd., Chicago, IL 60612
* Corresponding author.
E-mail address: estepanski@sosacorn.com (E.J. Stepanski).

doi:10.1016/j.jsmc.2006.11.011

Pittsburgh Sleep Quality Index, also found increased rates of abnormal sleep in cancer patients [2,11]. Application of stringent criteria appropriate to establish a formal diagnosis of insomnia as would be used by sleep specialists found that 19% of a sample of 300 women with nonmetastatic breast cancer who had received radiation therapy met criteria for an insomnia disorder [12].

In addition to these studies describing self-reported insomnia, a few studies using electroencephalogram (EEG)-based measures of sleep have documented decreased sleep quantity and quality among patients with cancer [14–16]. Savard and colleagues [16] found a baseline sleep efficiency of 82% with a total sleep time of about 6 hours in 57 patients with nonmetastatic breast cancer. A sleep efficiency of 78% has been reported in a sample of 72 patients with stage III or IV solid tumors taking opioids [14]. These patients also had decreased slow wave sleep (0.3%). Silberfarb and colleagues [15] found decreased sleep quantity and quality in lung cancer patients compared with breast cancer patients and control subjects.

Actigraphy has also been used as an objective measure of sleep in studies of patients with cancer [17–20]. A sleep efficiency of 71% was found using actigraphy in 24 patients undergoing radiation therapy for bone metastases [17]. Actigraphically measured sleep was shown to vary along with ratings of fatigue in patients through the course of chemotherapy [18,19].

Patients with cancer commonly report extreme daytime fatigue. As with poor sleep, increased fatigue is found before treatment [20], during chemotherapy [21], and for years after treatment is complete [22]. The prevalence of fatigue in this population is extremely high, with estimates as high as 92% of patients receiving chemotherapy [21]. Because the experience of fatigue is nearly universal, and because it is thought that this fatigue is etiologically distinct from other types of fatigue, the term "cancer-related fatigue" (CRF) is used to describe this phenomenon. The most commonly investigated cause of CRF is anemia. There is a large literature showing that chemotherapy-induced anemia correlates with CRF, and showing that CRF improves with successful treatment of anemia. This research also shows that anemia explains only part of the variance in fatigue scores [23]. Other proposed contributors to CRF include other chemotherapy effects [24], radiotherapy [25], inflammation [26], and mood [27]. The prevailing belief among cancer researchers has been that sleep disturbance is not an important determinant of CRF because it does not remit following nights of improved sleep. This impression is based on anecdotal clinical experience rather than controlled research.

Controlled studies show, as expected, that patients with worse sleep also report worse fatigue [20,27]. Therefore, even if poor sleep is not the primary factor contributing to CRF, it is one factor that should be accounted for when trying to understand all causes of CRF.

In general, research into CRF does not discriminate between fatigue and excessive daytime sleepiness, as is typically the case in sleep disorders research. Fatigue is captured by self-report measures, and some of these measures do include categories other than "fatigue" that would be expected to relate to excessive daytime sleepiness. For example, 41% of a sample of 527 cancer patients rated "drowsy" as a moderate or severe symptom [1]. This compared with 69% of this same sample rating "fatigue" as moderate or severe, suggesting that patients discriminated between these two symptoms. Another study found 60% of cancer patients endorsed "feeling drowsy" [3]. These results are provocative in that physiological sleepiness, at least in a subset of patients, may play a role in what has been categorized as CRF. Objective measures of sleepiness in these patients are needed to bring clarity to this issue.

Types and causes of sleep disturbance in cancer

Insomnia

The etiology of insomnia is presumably multifactorial, and hypothesized to be associated with psychological factors (eg, anxiety, depression), medical factors (eg, pain, chemotherapy-related toxicities), or behavioral factors (eg, decreased activity, increased time in bed, daytime napping). Traditional views of insomnia in a patient with cancer would assume that the insomnia is "secondary" to some aspect of the cancer. However, there has been a paradigm shift and current recommendations are that insomnia that accompanies a medical or psychiatric disorder is better understood as a comorbid disorder. The model of "comorbid insomnia" does not require an absolute linkage between the two disorders, and this is consistent with what has been reported regarding insomnia in patients with cancer. For example, a patient may begin to experience insomnia at the time of diagnosis, or in conjunction with chemotherapy, but the insomnia may persist for years following successful management of the cancer [12]. At that point, the insomnia is obviously an independent problem and requires focused treatment. The National Institutes of Health (NIH) state-of-the-science conference on insomnia in 2005 concluded that the traditional model of "secondary insomnia" leads to undertreatment of insomnia because of the often mistaken assumption that the insomnia would resolve with resolution of the primary condition [28]. This view of "comorbid" insomnia also fits with the trend in cancer research to view groups of frequently co-occurring symptoms as "symptom clusters" [29]. The study of symptom clusters recognizes that there are complex interrelationships between sets of symptoms—such as depression, pain, fatigue, and insomnia—that are not readily explained by unidirectional cause-and-effect models.

Pain

Increased pain has been shown to be related to sleep disturbance in patients with cancer [2,27,30]. This link between insomnia and pain in cancer patients is based on correlational data, and this is true of the scarce literature on sleep and pain generally. One recent exception is experimental data showing that sleep loss leads to increased pain [31]. Normal subjects who underwent partial sleep deprivation (4 hours time in bed) had significantly decreased pain thresholds the following day, as did patients who were exposed to interruption of rapid-eye movement (REM) sleep. The authors conclude that clinical conditions that cause decreased sleep time or interruption of REM sleep would be expected to contribute to increased pain. There is also a report showing that when sleep is improved in patients with pain (rheumatoid arthritis), the ratings of pain are improved as well [32]. Appreciation of this bidirectional relation between sleep and pain should inform clinical practice. While it is common to evaluate patients reporting persistent insomnia regarding their degree of pain control, it should also be the case that patients reporting significant pain be evaluated for adequacy of sleep. Optimal benefit may require intervention for both pain and sleep.

Psychological disturbance

In one report, 42% of a sample of 227 women with metastatic breast cancer were diagnosed with a psychiatric disorder [33]. The diagnosis was depression or anxiety in 36% of the sample. Psychological distress can be related to life-threatening illness as well as the treatment (eg, surgery, chemotherapy, radiotherapy).

Depressive symptoms occur commonly in conjunction with insomnia, particularly when comorbid medical illness is present [34]. High rates of depressive symptoms are found in cancer patients [35], and depression is closely associated with insomnia in this population [36]. It is known that the risk of depression is increased when chronic insomnia is present [37,38]. Depression has been shown to predict worse outcomes for cancer treatment, with increased mortality in patients with depression [39]. Therefore, it would be especially important to evaluate and treat insomnia in this population in an effort to decrease the risk of depression and poor outcome in the cancer treatment.

Behavioral factors

Patients struggling with cancer-related fatigue and pain are likely to decrease their activity level, and may go to bed earlier than they did in the past, or stay in bed later in the morning. Excessive time in bed is associated with insomnia. A second related behavior found in cancer patients that is problematic is the tendency to nap during the day. Studies of fatigue in cancer patients have found that patients with increased fatigue ratings were associated with decreased daytime activity and increased wakefulness at night [18,19]. Another study found that patients increased napping to 2 hours per day during chemotherapy [20]. Sleep during the day will displace sleep at night and can contribute to insomnia. If the napping is serving a therapeutic aim (eg, alleviating daytime fatigue/sleepiness, decreasing pain), patients may benefit from maintaining the napping, but should make the adjustment to a later bedtime to compensate for what will be a shorter nocturnal sleep period given the accumulation of daytime sleep.

Medication effects/toxicity

It is well documented that compounds used as anticancer agents—chemotherapy, immunotherapy, and other targeted therapies (eg, monoclonal antibodies)—are associated with significant toxicity to normal tissue. The specific toxicity profile, as well as the frequency and severity of these side effects, varies across compounds. Examples of adverse events of cancer treatments include neutropenia, thrombocytopenia, myelosuppression, cardiomyopathy, neuropathy, oral mucositis, diarrhea, nausea and vomiting, and alopecia. These toxicities can be both acute as well as chronic, with permanent damage occurring in some patients. Cognitive impairment has been demonstrated in breast cancer patients years after chemotherapy [40]. The term "chemobrain" has been used to refer to this cognitive impairment, and this may also be associated with fatigue, decreased QoL, and decreased mood [41]. Given the range of central nervous system (CNS) effects observed with these therapies, it is possible that sleep disturbance could result from CNS toxicity as a side effect of cancer treatment.

Cancer patients are also likely to receive many medications for supportive care, and these compounds may also have an adverse effect on sleep.

Specifically, opioid medication has been shown to significantly decrease the amount of slow wave sleep in normal sleepers with a single night of administration, compared with placebo [42]. Use of opioid medication has been hypothesized to contribute to observed increases in stage one non-rapid eye movement sleep in patients with cancer [14]. Opioid use may also contribute to increased sleep-disordered breathing, which would be expected to increase both reports of poor sleep quality and daytime impairment [43].

Another potential link between drug toxicity and poor sleep is through periodic limb movement disorder (PLMD). A study using polysomnography reported increased rates of PLMD in both breast and lung cancer patients [15]. Peripheral neuropathy is a risk factor for PLMD, and peripheral neuropathy is a dose-limiting toxicity for many anticancer agents [44,45].

Immune system function/inflammation

Several studies have shown changes in immune system function in response to experimental reductions in total sleep time [6,7]. Increased secretion of pro-inflammatory cytokines is found when sleep time is reduced in normal sleepers. Experimental reduction of total sleep time in normal sleepers does not produce the same behavioral effects as chronic insomnia, and therefore extrapolation of the effects of partial sleep deprivation to patients with insomnia on the rationale that both conditions are associated with decreased total sleep time is tenuous. However, patients with insomnia have also been shown to display differences in secretion of these cytokines, with increased secretion of interleukin (IL)-6 and tumor necrosis factor-alpha (TNF-α) during the day [46]. From this study, it is not possible to determine if the insomnia results from these cytokine abnormalities, or the other way around.

There is also research that demonstrates regulation of immune system function during normal sleep. This study found sleep-dependent regulation of immune function as opposed to showing abnormalities resulting from sleep loss [47]. This study assessed cytokine activity (I-12/I-10 ratio) in normal sleepers during sleep, as compared with during a night of total sleep deprivation. An increased I-12/I-10 ratio was found during the normal sleep condition, with no change in this measure during sustained wakefulness. This modulation of immune system function is hypothesized by the study authors to be sufficient to impact the course of disease in those disorders associated with type 2 cytokine overactivity. Classification of the immunological cytokines as type 1/type 2 is clinically useful as cytokines in each type tend to inhibit those in the other type. Type 2 cytokine overactivity is implicated in a number of autoimmune disorders, including HIV.

Chemotherapeutic agents are also capable of causing an inflammatory response [48], and it is possible that this is one mechanism producing poor sleep and fatigue in these patients. Changes in IL-6 have been shown to correlate with changes in fatigue in breast cancer patients undergoing chemotherapy [49]. Of interest, an intervention study using cognitive-behavioral therapy (CBT) to treat insomnia in cancer patients showed decreases in cytokines following successful treatment of insomnia [50].

Obstructive sleep apnea

The first report of sleep-disordered breathing associated with cancer is a case report from 1980 describing a patient with lymphocytic lymphoma with head and neck involvement [51]. The patient was found to have severe obstructive sleep apnea that was significantly improved, but not absent, following treatment for the lymphoma. Other recent studies have reported increased risk of sleep-disordered breathing in patients treated for head and neck cancer [52–54]. Payne and colleagues [53] prospectively assessed sleep in 17 patients with cancer of the oral cavity and oropharynx, and found an apnea-hypopnea index (AHI) greater than 20 in 13 of these patients, with a mean AHI of 44.7. Of note, the patients with obstructive sleep apnea (OSA) were more likely to have postsurgical complications, such as longer stays in the ICU and need for mechanical ventilation, compared with the non-OSA cohort. Friedman and colleagues [54] evaluated 24 patients who had completed surgical treatment for head and neck cancer, and found OSA (defined as an AHI >15) in 91.7%. These studies suggest that OSA is present at high levels both before and after treatment for head and neck cancer.

Treatment of insomnia in patients with cancer

The only intervention studies in cancer and insomnia employ behavioral treatment approaches in this population. Several investigators have shown positive results with the use of cognitive-behavioral therapy in the treatment of insomnia in patients with cancer [16,55–60]. These studies range from case series reports [55] to randomized controlled trials [16]. Also, a study that divided patients with early stage lung cancer into subgroups based on presence or absence of insomnia found evidence of the dysfunctional cognitive features typical of primary insomnia patients in the insomnia subgroup [27]. These include excessive rumination about the negative consequences of insomnia, as well as the expectation that their sleep can only improve with use of medication. These data show that cancer patients with insomnia display those features targeted by CBT, and therefore suggest that CBT may be an effective treatment in this population.

Behavioral treatment for patients with cancer

In 1983, Cannici and colleagues [56] tested progressive muscle relaxation training with a randomly selected group of 15 cancer patients with comorbid insomnia. Compared with 15 wait list controls, those receiving treatment had significantly reduced self-report sleep onset latencies at posttreatment and 3-month follow-up.

A study with 10 nonmetastatic breast cancer patients who received multicomponent CBT [57] also found significant improvements in sleep efficiency and total wake time that were sustained over time and substantiated with polysomnography. A similar multiple-case study [58] provided a 6-week behavioral group treatment program to 14 cancer patients. After 8 weeks these patients showed significant improvements in self-report of sleep efficiency, time awake after sleep onset, number of awakenings, and sleep quality ratings.

A quasi-experimental study with a heterogeneous group of cancer patients also provided support for the efficacy of behavioral treatment in this population. Simeit and colleagues [59] compared group multimodal behavioral treatment featuring progressive muscle relaxation (n = 80) and autogenic training (n = 71) to a nonrandomized convenience sample receiving various forms of standard care (n = 78). The two behavioral treatments led to self-report improvements in sleep latency, sleep quality, sleep medication use, and daytime dysfunction compared with controls.

Berger and colleagues [60] designed individualized programs with components of sleep hygiene, relaxation treatment, stimulus control, and sleep restriction for 21 breast cancer patients (stage I–II). Treatment for sleep followed four cycles of chemotherapy with doxorubicin. Sleep logs and actigraphy showed mixed results, with sleep efficiencies of 82% to 92%. Sleep latencies were less than 30 minutes, but awakenings and wake after sleep onset were higher than desired. Adherence to the treatment components was high for everything except stimulus control.

In the only randomized controlled trial of CBT for insomnia in this population, Savard and colleagues [16] randomly assigned 57 patients with breast cancer to CBT (n = 27) or a wait-list control group (n = 30). Patients had stage I–III breast cancer and were required to have completed therapy 1 month before study enrollment. Treatment consisted of eight weekly group sessions that included stimulus control therapy, sleep restriction therapy, cognitive therapy, sleep hygiene instructions, and fatigue management. There were significant improvements in self-reported sleep parameters, although polysomnography did not find the same magnitude of improvement in sleep parameters.

Taken together, these studies demonstrate that use of CBT for insomnia is effective in patients with nonmetastatic breast cancer. There are promising results in studies of mixed samples of cancer patients; however, results in those samples require replication in larger samples and in randomized controlled trials.

Chronomodulated chemotherapy

Another area where sleep and biological rhythms research may be important in the management of cancer is in determining the optimal timing of delivery of chemotherapy. Animal research has clearly shown a different pattern of toxicity with chemotherapy depending on the timing of the infusion [61]. The significance of this effect in human patients with cancer is unclear, with strong opinions on both sides of the issue appearing in the literature [62,63]. There is general agreement that toxicities can be lowered with chronomodulated chemotherapy, but disagreement about whether this translates into improved efficacy.

The current standard of care when applying chemotherapy is to infuse the cancer patient with chemotherapeutic agents at a fixed rate. However, there has been interest in potentially enhancing chemotherapy by exploiting circadian rhythms in the toxicity and antitumor efficacy of chemotherapy. Metastatic colorectal cancer has most typically been studied because of the relatively high incidence and poor outcome of this cancer. In treating this cancer, several studies have chronomodulated the administration of fluorouracil, leucovorin, and oxaliplatin.

The least toxic time for the administration of these drugs were initially determined from experiments in nocturnal rodents [61]. The time of administration was referenced to lights on, or the start of the rodent rest phase. The time of least toxicity was extrapolated to humans with reference to a typical bedtime of 23:00 [62]. For example, fluorouracil was found to be least toxic in mice 5 hours after lights on, which was estimated to be 04:00 in humans (23:00 + 5 hours). Similarly, the least toxic time for the administration of leucovorin to humans was estimated to be at 04:00 and for oxaliplatin at 16:00 [64].

In chronomodulated chemotherapy, the chemotherapeutic drugs are typically administered in a sinusoidal pattern over several hours, via the use of programmable multichannel pumps [65]. The concentration of each drug peaks at the estimated time of least toxicity. Typically the administration occurs over several days, repeating every few weeks. Because toxicity is lower, many studies increase the dose in an attempt to improve efficacy. After an initial visit to the hospital to be connected to the pump, patients have received chronomodulated chemotherapy at home or during usual activities [66].

The largest randomized trial of chronomodulated chemotherapy versus fixed rate infusion has recently been published [67], and avoids some of the design issues associated with two previous randomized trials (potential inactivation of the fixed rate infusions [68], crossover of fixed rate infusion patients into the chronomodulated group) [69]. Specifically this trial compared a 4-day chronomodulated treatment against a conventional 2-day fixed rate infusion. When individual patient toxicity permitted, doses of fluorouracil were escalated in both groups to a similar extent. In terms of toxicity incidence, neutropenia was three times more likely in the fixed rate infusion group, but diarrhea was three times more likely in the chronomodulated group. There was no statistically significant group difference in objective response rate or in median survival rate (18.7 months in the fixed rate infusion group, 19.6 months in the chronomodulated group). However, chronomodulated chemotherapy significantly increased survival rate in men by 3.1 months, but significantly decreased it by 2.8 months in women. It is not yet clear why this sex difference exists. These results illustrate that there is much to learn about circadian variation in these drug effects before optimal treatment plans can be designed.

Delivery of chronomodulated therapies will be easier as the number of effective oral agents used in cancer treatment increases. A recently published study investigated the regimen XELOX (oxaliplatin and capecitabine) as first-line treatment for metastatic colorectal cancer using a chronomodulated administration schedule for the capecitabine, an oral agent [70]. This phase II trial found a median time to progression of 9 months, and an overall survival of more than 24 months, both of which compare favorably to rates seen in prior phase II trials of XELOX. Additionally, the rates of toxicities were lower in this study. For example, the rate of grades 3 and 4 sensory neuropathy was reported as 2.2%, compared with historical rates with this regimen of 4% to 17%.

Importantly, chronomodulated chemotherapy is not simply altering the timing of chemotherapy, but often leads to a different sequence of drug exposure, intermittent administration, and increased duration of administration [63]. Thus, whether the timing of chemotherapy per se is responsible for the improved outcomes associated with chronomodulated chemotherapy remains to be determined. Large randomized trials supporting chronomodulated chemotherapy will be needed for it to significantly impact standard chemotherapy treatment in the United States. Nonetheless, the chronomodulated potential of other chemotherapeutic drug combinations may yield better outcomes than previous trials. For example, an increase in 10 months in the survival rate, to a median of 28 months, has recently been observed in colorectal patients with the chronomodulated administration of fluorouracil, leucovorin, and irinotecan [71]. Finally, chronomodulated chemotherapy may be enhanced by fine tuning its timing to individual circadian phase [72]. A reliable marker of circadian phase is the endogenous melatonin rhythm, which can be estimated via saliva or urine sampling at home [73].

Summary

Patients with cancer commonly report disturbed sleep, fatigue, and daytime drowsiness. Although sleep disturbance contributes to significantly reduced quality of life in patients with cancer, the overall significance of poor sleep as it relates to fatigue, pain, depression, or other health outcomes is unknown. Given that management of these symptoms is desirable for optimal outcomes in the treatment of cancer, evaluation and treatment of sleep disturbance in patients undergoing treatment for cancer is important. Given the need to minimize treatment burden, evaluation and treatment of sleep disturbance in this population may require clinical protocols specifically designed for patients with cancer. Further investigation is also needed into the role of pro-inflammatory cytokines as either a cause or consequence of sleep disturbance in this population.

References

[1] Cleeland CS, Mendoza TR, Wang XS, et al. Assessing symptom distress in cancer patients. Cancer 2000;89:1634–46.

[2] Fortner BV, Stepanski EJ, Wang SC, et al. Sleep and quality of life in breast cancer patients. J Pain Symptom Manage 2002;24:471–80.

[3] Portenoy RK, Thaler HT, Kornblith AB, et al. Symptom prevalence, characteristics and distress

in a cancer population. Qual Life Res 1994;3:
183–9.

[4] Berger AM, Sankaranarayanan J, Watanabe-
Galloway S. Current methodological approaches
to the study of sleep disturbances and quality of
life in adults with cancer: a systematic review.
Psychooncology, in press.

[5] Vena C, Parker K, Allen R, et al. Sleep-wake disturbances and quality of life in patients with
advanced lung cancer. Oncol Nurs Forum
2006;33:761–9.

[6] Redwine L, Hauger RL, Gillin JC, et al. Effects of
sleep and sleep deprivation on interleukin-6,
growth hormone, cortisol, and melatonin levels
in humans. J Clin Endocrinol Metab 2000;85:
3597–603.

[7] Vgontzas AN, Zoumakis M, Bixler EO, et al.
Adverse effects of modest sleep restriction on
sleepiness, performance, and inflammatory cytokines. J Clin Endocrinol Metab 2004;89:
2119–26.

[8] Krueger JM, Majde JA, Obal F. Sleep in host
defense. Brain Behav Immun 2003;17(Suppl 1):
S41–7.

[9] Davidson JR, MacLean AW, Brundage MD, et al.
Sleep disturbance in cancer patients. Soc Sci
Med 2002;54:1309–21.

[10] Koopman C, Nouriani B, Erickson V, et al. Sleep
disturbances in women with metastatic breast
cancer. Breast J 2002;8:362–70.

[11] Carpenter JS, Andrykowski MA. Psychometric
evaluation of the Pittsburgh Sleep Quality Index.
J Psychosom Res 1998;45:5–13.

[12] Savard J, Simard S, Blanchard J, et al. Prevalence,
clinical characteristics, and risk factors for insomnia in the context of breast cancer. Sleep
2001;24:583–90.

[13] Ohayon MM. Epidemiology of insomnia: what
we know and what we still need to learn. Sleep
Med Rev 2002;6:97–111.

[14] Parker KP, Bliwise DL, Dalton J, et al. Polysomnographic measures of sleep moderate the relationship between depression and pain. J Clin
Oncol 2006;24:474s [abstract].

[15] Silberfarb PM, Hauri PJ, Oxman PE, et al. Assessment of sleep in patients with lung cancer
and breast cancer. J Clin Oncol 1993;11:
997–1004.

[16] Savard J, Simard S, Ivers H, et al. Randomized
study on the efficacy of cognitive-behavioral
therapy for insomnia secondary to breast cancer,
part I: sleep and psychological effects. J Clin
Oncol 2005;23:6083–96.

[17] Miaskowski C, Lee KA. Pain, fatigue, and sleep
disturbances in oncology outpatients receiving
radiation therapy for bone metastasis: a pilot
study. J Pain Symptom Manage 1999;17:
320–32.

[18] Berger AM. Patterns of fatigue and activity and
rest during adjuvant breast cancer chemotherapy.
Oncol Nurs Forum 1998;25:51–62.

[19] Berger AM, Farr L. The influence of daytime inactivity and nighttime restlessness on cancer-related
fatigue. Oncol Nurs Forum 1999;26:1663–71.

[20] Ancoli-Israel S, Lui L, Marler MR, et al. Fatigue,
sleep, and circadian rhythms prior to chemotherapy for breast cancer. Support Care Cancer 2006;
14:201–9.

[21] Hartvig P, Aulin J, Hugerth M, et al. Fatigue in
cancer patients treated with cytotoxic drugs.
J Oncol Pharm Pract 2006;12:155–64.

[22] Goldstein D, Bennett B, Friedlander M, et al.
Fatigue states after cancer treatment occur both
in association with, and independent of, mood
disorder: a longitudinal study. BMC Cancer 2006;
6:240.

[23] Cella D, Lai JS, Chang CH, et al. Fatigue in cancer patients compared with fatigue in the general
United States population. Cancer 2002;94:
528–38.

[24] Jacobsen PB, Hann DM, Azzarello LM, et al. Fatigue in women receiving adjuvant chemotherapy for breast cancer: characteristics, course,
and correlates. J Pain Symptom Manage 1999;
18:235–42.

[25] Irvine DM, Vincent L, Graydon JE, et al. Fatigue
in women with breast cancer receiving radiation
therapy. Cancer Nurs 1998;21:127–35.

[26] Spath-Schwalbe E, Hansen K, Schmidt F, et al.
Acute effects of recombinant human interleu-
kin-6 on endocrine and central nervous sleep
functions in healthy men. J Clin Endocrinol
Metab 1998;83:1573–9.

[27] Rumble ME, Keefe FJ, Edinger JD, et al. A pilot
study investigating the utility of the cognitive-
behavioral model of insomnia in early-stage
lung cancer patients. J Pain Symptom Manage
2005;30:160–9.

[28] National Institutes of Health. National Institutes
of Health State of the Science Conference statement on Manifestations and Management of
Chronic Insomnia in Adults, June 13-15, 2005.
Sleep 2005;28:1049–57.

[29] Miaskowski C, Dodd M, Lee K. Symptom clusters: the new frontier in symptom management
research. J Natl Cancer Inst Monogr 2004;32:
17–21.

[30] Mercadante S, Girelli D, Casuccio A. Sleep disorders in advanced cancer patients: prevalence and
factors associated. Support Care Cancer 2004;12:
355–9.

[31] Roehrs T, Hyde M, Blaisdell B, et al. Sleep loss
and REM sleep loss are hyperalgesic. Sleep
2006;29:145–51.

[32] Schnitzer T, Rubens R, Wessel T, et al. The effect
of eszopiclone 3 mg compared with placebo in
patients with rheumatoid arthritis and co-exist-
ing insomnia. Sleep 2006;29:A238.

[33] Grabsch B, Clarke DM, Love A, et al. Psychological morbidity and quality of life in women with
advanced breast cancer: a cross-sectional survey.
Palliat Support Care 2006;4:47–56.

[34] Katz DA, McHorney CA. Clinical correlates of insomnia in patients with chronic illness. Arch Intern Med 1998;158:1099–107.

[35] Bottomley A. Depression in cancer patients: a literature review. Eur J Cancer Care 1998;7: 181–91.

[36] Redeker NS, Lev EL, Ruggiero J. Insomnia, fatigue, anxiety, depression, and quality of life of cancer patients undergoing chemotherapy. Scholarly Inquiry for Nursing Practice: An International Journal 2000;14:275–89.

[37] Ford DE, Kamerow DB. Epidemiologic study of sleep disturbances and psychiatric disorders: an opportunity for prevention. JAMA 1989;262: 1479–84.

[38] Breslau N, Roth T, Rosenthal L, et al. Sleep disturbance and psychiatric disorders: a longitudinal epidemiological study of young adults. Biol Psychiatry 1996;39:411–8.

[39] Temel JS, Jackson VA, Billings A, et al. The effect of depression on survival in patients with newly diagnosed advanced non-small cell lung cancer (NSCLC). J Clin Oncol 2006;24:470S.

[40] Schagen SB, Muller MJ, Boogerd W, et al. Late effects of adjuvant chemotherapy on cognitive function: a follow-up study in breast cancer patients. Ann Oncol 2002;13:1387–97.

[41] Tchen N, Juffs HG, Downie FP, et al. Cognitive function, fatigue, and menopausal symptoms in women receiving adjuvant chemotherapy for breast cancer. J Clin Oncol 2003;21:4175–83.

[42] Dimsdale JE, Norman D, DeJardin D, et al. The effect of opioids on sleep architecture. J Clin Sleep Med, in press.

[43] Farney RJ, Walker JM, Cloward TV, et al. Sleep-disordered breathing associated with long-term opioid therapy. Chest 2003;123:632–9.

[44] Leonard GD, Wright MA, Quinn MG, et al. Survey of oxaliplatin-associated neurotoxicity using an interview-based questionnaire in patients with metastatic colorectal cancer. BMC Cancer 2005. Available at: http://www.biomedcentral.com/1471-2407/5/116. Accessed November 2006.

[45] Richardson PG, Briemberg H, Jagannath S, et al. Frequency, characteristics, and reversibility of peripheral neuropathy during treatment of advanced multiple myeloma with bortezomib. J Clin Oncol 2006;24:3113–20.

[46] Vgontzas AN, Zoumakis M, Papanicolaou DA, et al. Chronic insomnia is associated with a shift of interleukin-6 and tumor necrosis factor secretion from nighttime to daytime. Metabolism 2002;51:887–92.

[47] Lange T, Dimitrov S, Fehm HL, et al. Shift of monocyte function toward cellular immunity during sleep. Arch Intern Med 2006;166: 1695–700.

[48] Wood LJ, Nail LM, Perrin NA, et al. The cancer chemotherapy drug etoposide (VP-16) induced proinflammatory cytokine production and sickness behavior-like symptoms in a mouse model of cancer chemotherapy-related symptoms. Biol Res Nurs 2006;8:157–69.

[49] Mills PJ, Parker B, Dimsdale JE, et al. The relationship between fatigue and quality of life and inflammation during anthracycline-based chemotherapy in breast cancer. Biol Psychol 2005; 69:85–96.

[50] Savard J, Simard S, Ivers H, et al. Randomized study on the efficacy of cognitive-behavioral therapy for insomnia secondary to breast cancer, part II: immunologic effects. J Clin Oncol 2005; 23:6097–106.

[51] Zorick F, Roth T, Kramer M, et al. Exacerbation of upper-airway sleep apnea by lymphocytic lymphoma. Chest 1980;77:689–90.

[52] Neese W, Hoekema A, Stegenga B, et al. Prevalence of obstructive sleep apnoea following head and neck cancer treatment: a cross-sectional study. Oral Oncol 2006;42:108–14.

[53] Payne RJ, Hier MP, Kost KM, et al. High prevalence of obstructive sleep apnea among patients with head and neck cancer. J Otolaryngol 2005; 34:304–11.

[54] Friedman M, Landsberg R, Pryor S, et al. The occurrence of sleep-disordered breathing among patients with head and neck cancer. Laryngoscope 2001;111:1917–9.

[55] Stam HJ, Bultz BD. The treatment of severe insomnia in a cancer patient. J Behav Ther Exp Psychiatry 1986;17:33–7.

[56] Cannici J, Malcolm R, Peek LA. Treatment of insomnia in cancer patients using muscle relaxation training. J Behav Ther Exp Psychiatry 1983; 14:251–6.

[57] Quesnel C, Savard J, Simard S, et al. Efficacy of cognitive-behavioral therapy for insomnia in women treated for nonmetastatic breast cancer. J Consult Clin Psychol 2003;71: 189–200.

[58] Davidson JR, Waisberg JL, Brundage MD, et al. Nonpharmacologic group treatment of insomnia: a preliminary study with cancer survivors. Psychooncology 2001;10:389–97.

[59] Simeit R, Deck R, Conta-Marx B. Sleep management training for cancer patients with insomnia. Support Care Cancer 2004;12:176–83.

[60] Berger AM, VonEssen S, Kuhn BR, et al. Adherence, sleep, and fatigue outcomes after adjuvant breast cancer chemotherapy: results of a feasibility intervention study. Oncol Nurs Forum 2003; 30:513–22.

[61] Burns ER, Beland SS. Effect of biological time on the determination of the LD50 of 5-fluorouracil in mice. Pharmacology 1984;28:296–300.

[62] Levi F. Chronotherapeutics: the relevance of timing in cancer therapy. Cancer Causes Control 2006;17:611–21.

[63] Takimoto CH. Chronomodulated chemotherapy for colorectal cancer: failing the test of time? Eur J Cancer 2006;42:574–81.

[64] Boughattas NA, Levi F, Fournier C, et al. Circadian rhythm in toxicities and tissue uptake of

1,2-diamminocyclohexane(trans-1)oxalatoplatinum(II) in mice. Cancer Res 1989;49:3362–8.

[65] Levi F. From circadian rhythms to cancer chronotherapeutics. Chronobiol Int 2002;19:1–19.

[66] Chevalier V, Cure H, Chollet P, et al. Author reply. J Clin Oncol 2002;20:3938–9.

[67] Giacchetti S, Bjarnason G, Garufi C, et al. Phase III trial comparing 4-day chronomodulated therapy versus 2-day conventional delivery of fluorouracil, leucovorin, and oxaliplatin as first-line chemotherapy of metastatic colorectal cancer: the European Organisation for Research and Treatment of Cancer Chronotherapy Group. J Clin Oncol 2006;24:3562–9.

[68] Levi FA, Zidani R, Vannetzel JM, et al. Chronomodulated versus fixed-infusion-rate delivery of ambulatory chemotherapy with oxaliplatin, fluorouracil, and folinic acid (leucovorin) in patients with colorectal cancer metastases: a randomized multi-institutional trial. J Natl Cancer Inst 1994; 86:1608–17.

[69] Levi F, Zidani R, Misset JL. Randomised multicentre trial of chronotherapy with oxaliplatin, fluorouracil, and folinic acid in metastatic colorectal cancer. International Organization for Cancer Chronotherapy. Lancet 1997;350: 681–6.

[70] Santini D, Vincenzi B, Schiavon G, et al. Chronomodulated administration of oxaliplatin plus capecitabine (XELOX) as first line chemotherapy in advanced colorectal cancer patients: phase II study. Cancer Chemother Pharmacol, in press.

[71] Garufi C, Vanni B, Aschelter AM, et al. Randomised phase II study of standard versus chronomodulated CPT-11 plus chronomodulated 5-fluorouracil and folinic acid in advanced colorectal cancer patients. Eur J Cancer 2006;42: 608–16.

[72] Hrushesky W, Wood P, Levi F, et al. A recent illustration of some essentials of circadian chronotherapy study design. J Clin Oncol 2004;22: 2971–2972; [author reply: 2972].

[73] Mundey K, Benloucif S, Harsanyi K, et al. Phase-dependent treatment of delayed sleep phase syndrome with melatonin. Sleep 2005;28: 1271–8.

SLEEP MEDICINE CLINICS

Sleep Med Clin 2 (2007) 77–86

Sleep, Blood Pressure Regulation, and Hypertension

Sean M. Caples, DO[a],*, Virend K. Somers, MD, DPhil[b,c]

- Blood pressure in normal sleep
  Nyctohemeral changes, sleep, and the autonomic nervous system
- Dippers versus non-dippers
- Interactions between sleep duration, hypertension, and systemic disease
- Obstructive sleep apnea
- Acute pathophysiologic mechanisms
- Potential mechanisms related to vascular pathology in obstructive sleep apnea
  Obstructive sleep apnea and systemic hypertension
- References

The link between sleep and the cardiovascular system is well recognized, both in health and disease. Because of the relative ease of noninvasive ambulatory measurement, no aspect of this relationship has been more studied than blood pressure (BP). The study of obstructive sleep apnea (OSA) has furthered the understanding of BP and its regulatory mechanisms, which are outlined in this article. More recently, as the scientific and public eyes have focused on inadequate sleep as a plague of modern society, research efforts have been directed at the consequences of sleep debt on systemic disease, including BP dysregulation.

Blood pressure in normal sleep

Nyctohemeral changes, sleep, and the autonomic nervous system

In normal individuals, sleep is associated with a reduced BP when compared with wakefulness. Referred to as the *dipping* phenomenon, systolic and diastolic BP may decline as much as 10% to 15% during sleep [1,2].

Several factors contribute to this circadian variation in BP. Autonomic neural influences play a key role. In humans, wakefulness normally transitions to non–rapid eye movement (NREM) sleep, which constitutes most of the sleep time and, compared with wakefulness, is characterized by cardiovascular stability. With parasympathetic predominance by way of sympathetic neural withdrawal, NREM is marked by a reduction in heart rate (HR) and BP. High baroreceptor gain maintains BP under tight control. Progression of NREM sleep from stage 1 through 4 is accompanied by further reduction in sympathetic neural traffic, so that by stages 3 and 4 (slow-wave), the output may be half that encountered in wakefulness [3,4]. Collectively, NREM is associated with lower BP, bradycardia, and reductions in cardiac output and systemic vascular resistance. Accordingly, serum catecholamines are at their lowest levels during sleep.

[a] Division of Pulmonary and Critical Care Medicine, Department of Medicine, Mayo Clinic, 200 First Street SW, Rochester, MN 55905, USA
[b] Division of Cardiovascular Diseases, Department of Medicine, Mayo Clinic, 200 First Street SW, Rochester, MN 55905, USA
[c] Division of Hypertension, Department of Medicine, Mayo Clinic, 200 First Street SW, Rochester, MN 55905, USA
* Corresponding author.
E-mail address: caples.sean@mayo.edu (S.M. Caples).

The stability of NREM is cyclically interrupted by rapid eye movement (REM) sleep, which occurs more frequently during the second half of the night. Phasic REM, defined by darting eye movements and skeletal muscle twitches, is associated with transient surges in sympathetic neural output, HR, and BP [4], the effects of which may be clinically important in individuals who have preexisting cardiovascular disease [5].

Physical and mental stress and activity contribute to higher BP during the day. Observational studies in humans show that less-active subjects have reduced daytime BP and therefore exhibit smaller relative dips in nocturnal BP [6]. The influence of body position is complex. Daytime maintenance of an upright posture through stimulation of cardiovascular reflexes results in autoregulatory increases in BP. However, the dipping pattern is also observed in individuals who maintain the supine position for 24 hours.

Studies incorporating sleep deprivation in healthy subjects suggest that although the reduction in nocturnal HR is maintained, the nocturnal BP drop is lost. This finding suggests that HR is largely influenced by the endogenous circadian clock, but BP may be linked more to the sleep–wake cycle, perhaps independently of circadian rhythm [7].

Dippers versus non-dippers

Dipping has been shown to blunt with aging, and differential effects may be present that are related to gender [8]. Race-dependent influences are suggested by less-pronounced dipping noted in studies of African Americans [9]. Individuals who have hypertension may exhibit dipping, but to a lesser extent than those who do not [8,10]. Studies comparing dippers with non-dippers have been limited somewhat by differing methods of measuring ambulatory BP and by varied applied definitions. However, population-based studies suggest heightened cardiovascular risk in non-dippers, who have been shown to have a higher risk for stroke [11] and incident heart failure [12], and that non-dipping is a risk factor for progression of renal disease [13]. These conditions are commonly comorbid with OSA, whose relationship with dipping is discussed later.

Furthermore, exaggerated (>20%) drops in BP during sleep, either induced by antihypertensive therapy or naturally in so-called "overdippers," may be a risk factor for target-organ ischemia in predisposed individuals, such as the elderly [14] and those who have coronary disease [15].

Interactions between sleep duration, hypertension, and systemic disease

Identified risk factors for hypertension include aging, obesity, and insulin resistance/hyperglycemia (often as part of the so-called "metabolic syndrome") [16,17], all of which have been associated with various sleep disorders, particularly OSA and chronic insomnia [18,19]. Thus, sleep and its derangements may be an important mediator, either directly or indirectly, in the development of hypertension. Admittedly, the interactions between these variables render disentangling the independent effects of sleep a challenge.

Intense interest has recently been focused on the downstream effects of short sleep duration on systemic health and disease. Central to this theme is the realization that members of western society lead progressively busier lives, obtain less sleep, and have increasing rates of obesity, hypertension, and cardiovascular disease [20,21]. Nightly sleep duration in the United States has dwindled by an estimated 2 hours over the past century. The National Sleep Foundation's Sleep in America poll reported that more than two thirds of the population obtains less than 8 hours of sleep per weeknight [22], a finding that may be partly explained by longer work days. Self-reporting of greater hours of work per week has been found to correlate with prevalent hypertension [23].

Proof of concept supporting the proposed role of sleep debt on these tangible systemic outcomes originates from human experiments of sleep deprivation, mostly in healthy subjects. The most notable report came from Spiegel and colleagues [24], who found that 2 days of curtailed sleep resulted in dysregulation of appetite hormones, accompanied by increased hunger and appetite. Admittedly, data from controlled laboratory-based sleep deprivation experiments in healthy volunteers are difficult to extrapolate to a larger population that may adapt over time to lifestyles that, to some extent, are chosen. However, recent longitudinal data from population based cohorts may help bridge this gap. The National Health and Nutrition Examination Survey I (NHANES I) showed that, over 10 years of follow-up of a middle-aged population, self-reported sleep of less than 7 hours per night was associated with higher body mass index and an increased likelihood of obesity compared with self-reported sleep of 7 or more hours [25]. Similar results have been seen in cohorts of younger adults and those in rural communities [26,27]. Positive associations reported between short sleep duration and glucose intolerance [28,29] may be directly related to mechanisms responsible for weight gain as outlined here.

Although the development of hypertension may be mediated largely through comorbid obesity, experimental and observational data implicate sleep debt as an independent risk factor for hypertension. This hypothesis is biologically plausible on several fronts. The cumulative BP load and exposure to an activated sympathetic nervous system is increased as time awake is prolonged, whereas the protective effects of reduced BP and sympathetic withdrawal during sleep are truncated [30].

Acute experimental restrictions on sleep in hypertensive and normotensive individuals have been associated with higher daytime BP. Some studies have shown increases in sympathetic neural activity, a finding that depends somewhat on the method through which autonomics are measured. Healthy individuals subjected to a single night of total sleep deprivation showed increased BP without attendant increases in heart rate or muscle sympathetic nervous activity, suggesting pressor effects independent of autonomic influences [31]. However, analysis of HR variability after short-term sleep restriction in healthy subjects suggested heightened sympathetic cardiac tone [32,33] associated with acute elevations in daytime BP. This finding occurred despite disproportionate reductions in recorded REM sleep [33], the loss of which may be expected to reduce overall sympathetic output. Increases in urinary catecholamines suggested heightened sympathetic output associated with elevated BP and HR in patients who had untreated hypertension after a single night of sleep deprivation [34].

Very recently published longitudinal, population-based studies are bolstering the relationship between sleep and hypertension. Gangwisch and colleagues [35] again used NHANES I data to show significant increases in incident hypertension over 10 years in those who reported sleep durations of 5 hours or less per night. This relationship was minimally attenuated after controlling for obesity and diabetes. In the cross-sectional Sleep Heart Health Study, the highest odds of hypertension were seen in those reporting less than 6 hours per night [36]. Reporting more than 8 to 9 hours per night also conferred a higher risk for hypertension, although lower than in those who had the shortest sleep duration.

Some observational reports have suggested an association between increased mortality and short sleep duration [37,38], a link that is plausibly mediated by hypertension. Other potential modifiers include the association between short sleep and coronary disease as reported from the Nurses Health Study [28] and the finding that sleep restriction in healthy individuals is associated with increased serum levels of C-reactive protein [39], an inflammatory marker directly associated with heightened cardiovascular mortality [40].

Results from observational studies, however, are not consistent regarding self-reported short sleep duration and cardiovascular outcomes. Analysis of questionnaires from more than 1 million respondents showed the most favorable mortality rates in those reporting 7 hours of sleep per night, with slightly higher risk attributable to longer sleep durations [41]. This study also focused on complaints of insomnia, which did not contribute to risk. Methodological limitations notwithstanding, this finding may underscore mechanisms of insomnia that are pathophysiologically distinct from volitional short sleep or may relate to sleep-time misperceptions common in those who have insomnia [42].

An important caveat regarding these data linking sleep duration and disease outcomes is the low level of evidence afforded by self-report questionnaires. Despite large numbers of subjects, this methodology presents the potential for several inherent biases, particularly considering that sleep time misperception is common. Only recently have longitudinal observational studies suggested a more durable proof of concept, but again by way of self-reporting. To more fully determine cause and effect, rigorous and undoubtedly expensive interventional controlled trials may be needed.

Further study is also needed to guide treatment recommendations. Drug treatment for hypertension is well known to reduce mortality [43]. Given the lack of well-designed interventional trials, whether targeted lowering of nocturnal BP, either in dippers or non-dippers, affords any further benefit over antihypertensive therapy in general is unclear. Drug treatment trials assessing overnight BP, many of which were uncontrolled, have not adequately addressed this question [14,44,45]. Given the potential risk attributable to exaggerated lowering of nocturnal BP, further guidance is needed. The importance of nonpharmacologic treatment of hypertension also requires that future studies incorporate and assess measures that may impact nocturnal BP. Finally, obtaining more sleep on a nightly basis has many potential benefits, as some blanket statements recommend. However, further study of potential mechanisms to explain the association between increased mortality and excessively long sleep duration should be undertaken. The physiologic underpinnings of optimal sleep time, a widely variable parameter among individuals, are poorly understood.

Obstructive sleep apnea

OSA is characterized by repetitive episodes of upper airway narrowing or occlusion that cause acute stressors, such as hypoxemia and reoxygenation, swings in intrathoracic pressure, and central nervous system (CNS) arousals. Apneic events are associated with well-recognized acute increases in peripheral vasoconstriction and attendant rises in BP during sleep. Accumulating evidence in humans supports a probable causative role for OSA in diurnal hypertension. Data on the impact of OSA treatment on BP, particularly with continuous positive airway pressure (CPAP) therapy, are accumulating but not always consistent.

Acute pathophysiologic mechanisms

Episodic deoxygenation drives many aspects of the acute and chronic pathophysiology of OSA. Hypoxemia stimulates the peripheral arterial chemoreceptors, the most important of which are the carotid bodies, and the responses of which are important in mediating the response to OSA-associated hypoxemia. Carotid body afferents, relaying in the brain stem, elicit reflex increases in sympathetic efferent traffic during hypoxemic stimulation, as shown by direct peripheral intraneural electrode recordings [46,47]. Stimulation of respiratory centers within the brainstem normally increases respiratory muscle output and minute ventilation. Under normal conditions, lung inflation, by way of stimulation of parenchymal vagal mechanoreceptors, tempers sympathetic outflow. The lack of lung inflation during apneas results in disinhibition of sympathetic neural activity, and therefore a potentiated sympathetic response to hypoxemia [4,48,49].

Individuals who have sleep apnea also seem to have an exaggerated peripheral chemoreflex response to hypoxemia, as shown by an augmented ventilatory and autonomic drive compared with nonapneic controls [50]. Chemoreflex activation results in increased sympathetic traffic to the peripheral vasculature, with a consequent acute rise in arterial BP [50,51]. This heightened chemoreflex sensitivity may contribute to enhanced sympathetic tone in OSA, even during normoxic wakefulness.

Homeostatic mechanisms, which under normal conditions temper increased sympathetic drive, are disrupted in OSA. In addition to the loss of vagal mechanisms related to reduced lung inflation during apnea, baroreflex dysfunction has also been identified in OSA. Originating in major blood vessels, such as in the carotid sinus and aorta, and mediated through the CNS, the baroreflexes also buffer ventilatory, pressor, and sympathetic responses to peripheral chemoreflex excitation [47,52]. Preexisting hypertension, often associated with OSA, may result in impaired baroreflex function and may therefore contribute indirectly to augmentation of the chemoreflex-mediated sympathetic response [53].

Repetitive breathing events in OSA commonly terminate in a CNS arousal, with restoration of upper airway patency and resumption of ventilation. Each arousal from sleep is accompanied by acute increases in sympathetic neural output [54] that may contribute to autonomic dysregulation characteristic of OSA.

Potential mechanisms related to vascular pathology in obstructive sleep apnea

Cumulative effects are probably related to the repetitive acute perturbations, which over time may be important in the pathogenesis of chronic conditions such as hypertension. Disturbed neural circulatory control during daytime wakefulness in patients who have OSA, even in the absence of overt vascular disease, is evident by the finding of heightened sympathetic drive through measurement of muscle sympathetic nervous activity, even in the absence of hypoxemia [51]. This finding may reasonably be attributable to increased tonic chemoreflex drive [55].

Abnormalities in HR and BP variability are present in OSA [56], which may be markers for future cardiovascular disease [57]. The vascular endothelium, a biologically active system, may also be dysfunctional in OSA. Whether this results from OSA per se is not entirely clear, but large population-based studies suggest that endothelial dysfunction may be an important marker of cardiovascular risk. The small-vessel dilatory response to vasoactive substances such as acetylcholine, which represents resistance vessel endothelial function, is blunted in sleep apnea [58,59], although these findings are not evident in all studies [60]. Whether large or conduit vessel endothelial function is also attenuated in OSA is unclear. Levels of serum endothelin, a potent vasoconstrictor, may also be elevated in patients who have OSA compared with control subjects [61].

Other features of OSA may indirectly increase the risk for hypertension, including the striking prevalence of overweight and obesity, which are primary risk factors in this patient population. Although excess body weight independently puts these patients at risk for diabetes, other mechanisms in OSA contribute to glucose intolerance, including increased sympathetic tone, repetitive hypoxemia, and sleep debt. Clinic- and population-based studies [62,63], mostly of men who have severe OSA, support a relationship independent of obesity [64]. OSA treatment trials have shown mild and short-lived results in the reversal of glucose intolerance [65]. Heightened inflammation, as shown by elevated biomarkers such as C-reactive protein, may also modulate vascular risk in patients who have

OSA. Research at the cellular level further supports this theory. Up-regulation of leukocyte adhesion factors in OSA [66,67], although not yet proven to translate to clinical disease, could predispose to endothelial injury and vascular events. These pathways could be mediated through neutrophil-derived oxidative stress [68] and abnormalities in coagulation markers in patients who have OSA [69].

Evidence supports the role of reduced levels of the potent vasodilator nitric oxide in mediating vascular disease and BP regulation in OSA. Ip and colleagues [70] found significant correlations between reduced nitrite and nitrate levels and severity of OSA, with significant increases in these levels after overnight application of CPAP.

Hypoxia is known to stimulate vascular endothelial growth factors (VEGF), which are elevated in OSA [71,72]. One year of CPAP use is associated with reductions in VEGF levels compared with those of patients who are untreated [71]. Although direct evidence for stimulation of vascular growth through these proteins in OSA is currently lacking, promotion of neovascularization and proliferative mechanisms could represent adaptive mechanisms in OSA, with implications for understanding the end-organ effects of repetitive hypoxia.

Obstructive sleep apnea and systemic hypertension

Observational studies have shown that hypertension and OSA often coexist and that individuals who have sleep apnea tend to have higher BPs than matched controls. These individuals also have less BP dipping at night (Fig. 1), which may itself confer added cardiovascular risk [73].

Despite the strong association between OSA and hypertension, the challenges of identifying any independent causative role for OSA in hypertension must be acknowledged. Both conditions are exceedingly common, are more prevalent with aging, and often coexist not only together but also in concert with other comorbidities that confer their own risk for vascular disease, such as obesity and glucose intolerance. The literature has been dominated by case-control studies with their attendant biases. Finally, because OSA severity continues to be characterized by the apnea–hypopnea index (AHI), the relative effects of potentially important non–frequency-based parameters, such as duration and degree of hypoxemia, are probably under-recognized.

Early cross-sectional reports linking OSA and systemic hypertension were limited by study design and potentially confounding effects of comorbid variables, particularly obesity. Nevertheless, these reports provided an important basis for subsequent confirmation by more comprehensive population-based studies. Although these prevalence data showed an association between OSA and hypertension [74,75], they lacked longitudinal observation to implicate causality. A prospective study from the Wisconsin Sleep Cohort provided persuasive evidence implicating OSA as a possible causal factor in hypertension [74]. Specifically, the presence of hypertension 4 years after initial assessment was found to depend on the severity of OSA at baseline. However, the study did not specifically identify

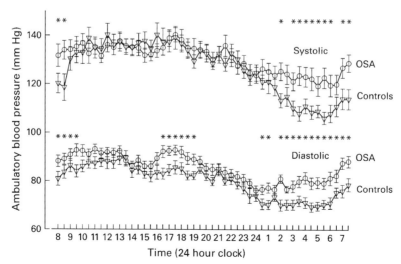

Fig. 1. Twenty-four–hour systolic and diastolic BP profiles for patients who have OSA and controls matched for age, body mass index, and treatment for hypertension, among other variables. Note less dipping at night and higher diastolic BP over the later afternoon hours in the OSA group. (*From* Davies CWH, Crosby JH, Mullins RL, et al. Case control study of 24 hour ambulatory blood pressure in patients with obstructive sleep apnoea and normal matched control subjects. Thorax 2000;55(9):736–40; with permission from the BMJ Publishing Group.)

subjects free of hypertension at baseline and could not determine the incident risk imparted by OSA. Further shortcomings included the 10% of patients at baseline and 17% at follow-up who were treated with antihypertensive medications. Post-hoc analysis excluding those who had hypertension or taking antihypertensives at baseline resulted in similar associations between AHI and hypertension at 4-year follow-up [76]. Collectively, available data implicate OSA not only in acute increases in nocturnal BP but also in sustained daytime hypertension.

CPAP, which is the most effective therapy for OSA, has been shown to acutely attenuate sympathetic drive and nocturnal BP in patients who have OSA [51,77,78]. However, data regarding effects on daytime BP have been more difficult to interpret. Several observational studies, often uncontrolled and from highly select populations, have suggested improvements in daytime BP control with the use of CPAP. Because of these shortcomings and an apparent true placebo effect realized in measurement of BP, several randomized, placebo-controlled studies have been performed and have yielded variable results. The generalizability of the studies are limited, because they comprise

small sample sizes and most subjects were normotensive at baseline.

However, some findings are notable. In the largest study to date, Pepperell and colleagues [79] found a small but significant reduction in BP in a largely normotensive cohort over only 4 weeks of therapy. Becker and colleagues [80], in a controlled trial comparing therapeutic with subtherapeutic CPAP, found fairly dramatic reductions in mean BP (9.9 ± 11.4 mm Hg) in a small cohort that had severe OSA (mean AHI>60/h) treated for more than 60 days, which is the longest trial to date (Fig. 2). Potential limitations of the study include a high dropout rate and the fact that approximately two thirds were treated with various antihypertensive medications. Subtherapeutic CPAP reduced the AHI by 50% but did not result in any reduction in BP, suggesting the importance of treatment dose–effect.

A high prevalence of OSA is seen in hypertensive nondippers [81]. Although these patients may be more resistant to antihypertensive drug therapy, a small study from Edinburgh suggests that they may be more sensitive to the BP-reducing effects of nocturnal CPAP [82].

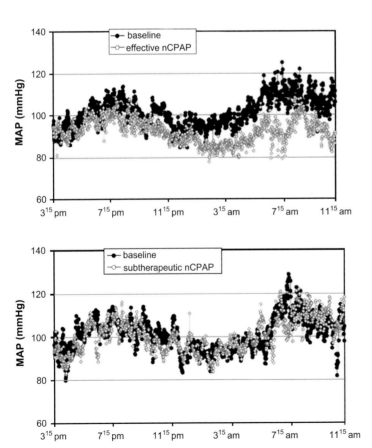

Fig. 2. BP profiles at baseline (*solid circles*) and after treatment with therapeutic (*upper box, open circles*) or subtherapeutic (*lower box, open circles*) CPAP in a small group of patients (mostly men) who have severe OSA (mean AHI>60). Most of the subjects were on drug treatment for hypertension. *Abbreviations:* MAP, mean arterial pressure; nCPAP, nasal continuous positive airway pressure. (*From* Becker HF, Jerrentrup A, Ploch T, et al. Effect of nasal continuous positive airway pressure treatment on blood pressure in patients with obstructive sleep apnea. Circulation 2003;107(1):68–73; with permission.)

Although excessive daytime sleepiness is a common and potentially dangerous sequela of OSA, it is not a universal symptom. Increasing evidence suggests that sleepiness may be an important mediator of some of the systemic effects of OSA. That is, in the absence of sleepiness, even severe OSA as quantified by the AHI does not always translate to reductions in BP after CPAP treatment, regardless of whether normotension or hypertension exists at baseline. In a randomized controlled trial, Barbe and colleagues [83] showed that in normotensive individuals who had severe sleep apnea according to AHI criteria, but no daytime sleepiness, CPAP treatment imparted no reductions in BP. The Oxford group recently reported similar findings, but in a cohort of individuals who had hypertension and sleep apnea [84]. Even mild subjective sleepiness confers some BP benefit with the use of CPAP [85].

Finally, a recent randomized trial compared ambulatory BP in individuals who had moderately severe sleep apnea after treatment with therapeutic CPAP, sham CPAP, or supplemental oxygen [86]. Although therapeutic CPAP resulted in BP reductions, supplemental oxygen did not, despite normalizing oxygen saturation. This finding suggests that hypoxia-mediated mechanisms may not fully explain the acute and chronic effects of sleep apnea on the vasculature. Therefore, CNS arousals, which are attenuated, if not abolished, with CPAP therapy, may be just as important, perhaps by way of effects on sympathetic output or hemodynamics.

Because chronic conditions such as OSA-associated hypertension could reasonably lead to vascular remodeling and other structural cardiovascular changes, short-term controlled studies may fail to disclose the true effects of consistent CPAP therapy on hypertension and its consequences. Furthermore, given the prevalence of hypertension and its effects on the development of other cardiovascular disease, including heart failure and stroke, the results of small changes in BP and decreases in nocturnal BP may be far-reaching.

References

[1] Staessen J, Bulpitt CJ, O'Brien E, et al. The diurnal blood pressure profile. A population study. Am J Hypertens 1992;5(6 I):386–92.

[2] Staessen JA, Fagard RH, Lijnen PJ, et al. Mean and range of the ambulatory pressure in normotensive subjects from a meta-analysis of 23 studies. Am J Cardiol 1991;67(8):723–7.

[3] Hornyak M, Cejnar M, Elam M, et al. Sympathetic muscle nerve activity during sleep in man. Brain 1991;114(3):1281–95.

[4] Somers VK, Dyken ME, Mark AL, et al. Sympathetic-nerve activity during sleep in normal subjects. N Engl J Med 1993;328(5):303–7.

[5] Verrier RL, Muller JE, Hobson JA. Sleep, dreams, and sudden death: the case for sleep as an autonomic stress test for the heart. Cardiovasc Res 1996;31(2):181–211.

[6] O'Shea JC, Murphy MB. Nocturnal blood pressure dipping: a consequence of diurnal physical activity blipping? Am J Hypertens 2000;13(6):601–6.

[7] Kerkhof GA, Van Dongen HPA, Bobbert AC. Absence of endogenous circadian rhythmicity in blood pressure? Am J Hypertens 1998;11(3 I):373–7.

[8] Verdecchia P, Porcellati C, Schillaci G, et al. Ambulatory blood pressure. An independent predictor of prognosis in essential hypertension [published erratum appears in Hypertension 1995 Mar;25(3):462]. Hypertension 1994;24(6):793–801.

[9] Ancoli-Israel S, Stepnowsky C, Dimsdale J, et al. The effect of race and sleep-disordered breathing on nocturnal BP "dipping": analysis in an older population. Chest 2002;122(4):1148–55.

[10] Millar-Craig M, Bishop C, Raftery EB. Circadian variation of blood-pressure. Lancet 1978;311(8068):795–7.

[11] O'Brien E, Sheridan J, O'Malley K. Dippers and non-dippers. Lancet 1988;332(8607):397.

[12] Ingelsson E, Bjorklund-Bodegard K, Lind L, et al. Diurnal blood pressure pattern and risk of congestive heart failure. JAMA 2006;295(24):2859–66.

[13] Timio M, Venanzi S, Lolli S, et al. "Non-dipper" hypertensive patients and progressive renal insufficiency: a 3-year longitudinal study. Clin Nephrol 1995;43(6):382–7.

[14] Kario K, Pickering TG. Does extreme dipping of nocturnal blood pressure in elderly hypertensive patients confer high risk of developing ischemic target organ damage from antihypertensive therapy? Arch Intern Med 2000;160(9):1378.

[15] Pierdomenico S, Bucci A, Costantini F, et al. Circadian blood pressure changes and myocardial ischemia in hypertensive patients with coronary artery disease. J Am Coll Cardiol 1998;31(7):1627–34.

[16] Wilson PW, D'Agostino RB, Sullivan L, et al. Overweight and obesity as determinants of cardiovascular risk: the Framingham experience. Arch Intern Med 2002;162(16):1867–72.

[17] Sonne-Holm S, Sorensen TI, Jensen G, et al. Independent effects of weight change and attained body weight on prevalence of arterial hypertension in obese and non-obese men. BMJ 1989;299(6702):767–70.

[18] Caples SM, Gami AS, Somers VK. Obstructive sleep apnea. Ann Intern Med 2005;142(3):187–97.

[19] National Institutes of Health state of the science conference statement: manifestations and

management of chronic insomnia in adults June 13–15, 2005. Sleep 2005;28(9):1049–57.

[20] Kuczmarski RJ, Flegal KM, Campbell SM, et al. Increasing prevalence of overweight among US adults. The National Health and Nutrition Examination Surveys, 1960 to 1991. JAMA 1994;272(3):205–11.

[21] Hajjar I, Kotchen TA. Trends in prevalence, awareness, treatment, and control of hypertension in the United States, 1988–2000. JAMA 2003;290(2):199–206.

[22] National Sleep Foundation 2002 "Sleep in America" Poll; 2002 Available at: http://www.sleep foundation.org/_content/hottopics/2002SleepIn AmericaPoll.pdf. Accessed December 2006.

[23] Yang H, Schnall PL, Jauregui M, et al. Work hours and self-reported hypertension among working people in California. Hypertension 2006;48(4):744–50.

[24] Spiegel K, Tasali E, Penev P, et al. Brief communication: sleep curtailment in healthy young men is associated with decreased leptin levels, elevated ghrelin levels, and increased hunger and appetite. Ann Intern Med 2004;141(11):846–50.

[25] Gangwisch JE, Malaspina D, Boden-Albala B, et al. Inadequate sleep as a risk factor for obesity: analyses of the NHANES I. Sleep 2005;28(10):1289–96.

[26] Hasler G, Buysse DJ, Klaghofer R, et al. The association between short sleep duration and obesity in young adults: a 13-year prospective study. Sleep 2004;27(4):661–6.

[27] Kohatsu ND, Tsai R, Young T, et al. Sleep duration and body mass index in a rural population. Arch Intern Med 2006;166(16):1701–5.

[28] Ayas NT, White DP, Al-Delaimy WK, et al. A prospective study of self-reported sleep duration and incident diabetes in women. Diabetes Care 2003;26(2):380–4.

[29] Gottlieb DJ, Punjabi NM, Newman AB, et al. Association of sleep time with diabetes mellitus and impaired glucose tolerance. Arch Intern Med 2005;165(8):863–8.

[30] Egan BM. Sleep and hypertension: burning the candle at both ends really is hazardous to your health. Hypertension 2006;47(5):816–7.

[31] Kato M, Phillips BG, Sigurdsson G, et al. Effects of sleep deprivation on neural circulatory control. Hypertension 2000;35(5):1173–5.

[32] Tochikubo O, Ikeda A, Miyajima E, et al. Effects of insufficient sleep on blood pressure monitored by a new multibiomedical recorder. Hypertension 1996;27(6):1318–24.

[33] Spiegel K, Leproult R, Van Cauter E. Impact of sleep debt on metabolic and endocrine function. Lancet 1999;354(9188):1435–9.

[34] Lusardi P, Zoppi A, Preti P, et al. Effects of insufficient sleep on blood pressure in hypertensive patients: a 24-h study. Am J Hypertens 1999;12(1 Pt 1):63–8.

[35] Gangwisch JE, Heymsfield SB, Boden-Albala B, et al. Short sleep duration as a risk factor for

[36] Gottlieb DJ, Redline S, Nieto FJ, et al. Association of usual sleep duration with hypertension: the Sleep Heart Health Study. Sleep 2006;29(8):1009–14.

[37] Enstrom JE, Kanim LE, Breslow L. The relationship between vitamin C intake, general health practices, and mortality in Alameda County, California. Am J Public Health 1986;76(9):1124–30.

[38] Patel SR, Ayas NT, Malhotra MR, et al. A prospective study of sleep duration and mortality risk in women. Sleep 2004;27(3):440–4.

[39] Meier-Ewert HK, Ridker PM, Rifai N, et al. Effect of sleep loss on C-Reactive protein, an inflammatory marker of cardiovascular risk. J Am Coll Cardiol 2004;43(4):678–83.

[40] Ridker PM, Rifai N, Rose L, et al. Comparison of C-reactive protein and low-density lipoprotein cholesterol levels in the prediction of first cardiovascular events. N Engl J Med 2002;347(20):1557–65.

[41] Kripke DF, Garfinkel L, Wingard DL, et al. Mortality associated with sleep duration and insomnia. Arch Gen Psychiatry 2002;59(2):131–6.

[42] Edinger JD, Fins AI. The distribution and clinical significance of sleep time misperceptions among insomniacs. Sleep 1995;18(4):232–9.

[43] Staessen JA, Wang J-G, Thijs L. Cardiovascular protection and blood pressure reduction: a meta-analysis. Lancet 2001;358(9290):1305–15.

[44] White WB, Mehrotra DV, Black HR, et al. Effects of controlled-onset extended-release verapamil on nocturnal blood pressure (dippers versus nondippers). COER-Verapamil Study Group. Am J Cardiol 1997;80(4):469–74.

[45] Kohno I, Iwasaki H, Okutani M, et al. Administration-time-dependent effects of diltiazem on the 24-hour blood pressure profile of essential hypertension patients. Chronobiol Int 1997;14(1):71–84.

[46] Valbo ABHK, Torebjork HE, Wallin BG. Somatosensory, proprioceptive, and sympathetic activity in human peripheral nerves. Physiol Rev 1979;59:919–57.

[47] Somers V, Mark A, Abboud F. Interaction of baroreceptor and chemoreceptor control of sympathetic nerve activity in normal humans. J Clin Invest 1991;87:1953–7.

[48] Somers VK, Mark AL, Zavala DC, et al. Influence of ventilation and hypocapnia on sympathetic nerve responses to hypoxia in normal humans. J Appl Physiol 1989;67(5):2095–100.

[49] Smith ML, Niedermaier ONW, Hardy SM, et al. Role of hypoxemia in sleep apnea-induced sympathoexcitation. J Auton Nerv Syst 1996;56(3):184–90.

[50] Narkiewicz K, van de Borne PJH, Pesek CA, et al. Selective potentiation of peripheral chemoreflex sensitivity in obstructive sleep apnea. Circulation 1999;99(9):1183–9.

[51] Somers VK, Dyken ME, Clary MP, et al. Sympathetic neural mechanisms in obstructive sleep apnea. J Clin Invest 1995;96(4):1897–904.

[52] Heistad D, Abboud F, Mark A, et al. Interaction of baroreceptor and chemoreceptor reflexes. Modulation of chemoreceptor reflex by changes in baroreceptor activity. J Clin Invest 1974;53:1226–36.

[53] Hedner J, Wilcox I, Laks L, et al. A specific and potent pressor effect of hypoxia in patients with sleep apnea. Am Rev Respir Dis 1992;146: 1240–5.

[54] Blasi A, Jo J, Valladares E, et al. Cardiovascular variability after arousal from sleep: time-varying spectral analysis. J Appl Physiol 2003;95(4): 1394–404.

[55] Narkiewicz K, van de Borne PJ, Montano N, et al. Contribution of tonic chemoreflex activation to sympathetic activity and blood pressure in patients with obstructive sleep apnea. Circulation 1998;97(10):943–5.

[56] Narkiewicz K, Montano N, Cogliati C, et al. Altered cardiovascular variability in obstructive sleep apnea. Circulation 1998;98(11):1071–7.

[57] Tsuji H, Larson MG, Venditti FJ Jr, et al. Impact of reduced heart rate variability on risk for cardiac events. The Framingham Heart Study. Circulation 1996;94(11):2850–5.

[58] Kato M, Roberts-Thomson P, Phillips B. Impairment of endothelium-dependent vasodilation of resistance vessels in patients with obstructive sleep apnea. Circulation 2000;102:2607–10.

[59] Carlson J, Rangemark C, Hedner J. Attenuated endothelium-dependent vascular relaxation in patients with sleep apnoea. J Hypertens 1996; 14:577–84.

[60] Kraiczi H, Hedner J, Peker Y, et al. Increased vasoconstrictor sensitivity in obstructive sleep apnea. J Appl Physiol 2000;89(2):493–8.

[61] Phillips BG, Narkiewicz K, Pesek CA, et al. Effects of obstructive sleep apnea on endothelin-1 and blood pressure. J Hypertens 1999;17(1):61–6.

[62] Punjabi NM, Sorkin JD, Katzel LI, et al. Sleep-disordered breathing and insulin resistance in middle-aged and overweight men. Am J Respir Crit Care Med 2002;165(5):677–82.

[63] Ip MS, Lam B, Ng MM, et al. Obstructive sleep apnea is independently associated with insulin resistance. Am J Respir Crit Care Med 2002; 165(5):670–6.

[64] Punjabi NM, Ahmed MM, Polotsky VY, et al. Sleep-disordered breathing, glucose intolerance, and insulin resistance. Respir Physiol Neurobiol 2003;136(2–3):167–78.

[65] Harsch IA, Schahin SP, Radespiel-Troger M, et al. Continuous positive airway pressure treatment rapidly improves insulin sensitivity in patients with obstructive sleep apnea syndrome. Am J Respir Crit Care Med 2004;169(2):156–62.

[66] Lavie L, Vishnevsky A, Lavie P. Evidence for lipid peroxidation in obstructive sleep apnea. Sleep 2004;27(1):123–8.

[67] Dyugovskaya L, Lavie P, Lavie L. Increased adhesion molecules expression and production of reactive oxygen species in leukocytes of sleep apnea patients. Am J Respir Crit Care Med 2002;165(7):934–9.

[68] Schulz R, Mahmoudi S, Hattar K, et al. Enhanced release of superoxide from polymorphonuclear neutrophils in obstructive sleep apnea. Impact of continuous positive airway pressure therapy. Am J Respir Crit Care Med 2000;162(2):566–70.

[69] von Kanel R, Dimsdale JE. Hemostatic alterations in patients with obstructive sleep apnea and the implications for cardiovascular disease. Chest 2003;124(5):1956–67.

[70] Ip MSM, Lam B, Chan L-Y, et al. Circulating nitric oxide is suppressed in obstructive sleep apnea and is reversed by nasal continuous positive airway pressure. Am J Respir Crit Care Med 2000;162(6):2166–71.

[71] Lavie L, Kraiczi H, Hefetz A, et al. Plasma vascular endothelial growth factor in sleep apnea syndrome: effects of nasal continuous positive air pressure treatment. Am J Respir Crit Care Med 2002;165(12):1624–8.

[72] Schulz R, Hummel C, Heinemann S, et al. Serum levels of vascular endothelial growth factor are elevated in patients with obstructive sleep apnea and severe nighttime hypoxia. Am J Respir Crit Care Med 2002;165(1):67–70.

[73] Davies CWH, Crosby JH, Mullins RL, et al. Case-control study of 24 hour ambulatory blood pressure in patients with obstructive sleep apnoea and normal matched control subjects. Thorax 2000;55(9):736–40.

[74] Peppard PE, Young T, Palta M, et al. Prospective study of the association between sleep-disordered breathing and hypertension. N Engl J Med 2000;342(19):1378–84.

[75] Young T, Peppard PE, Gottlieb DJ. Epidemiology of obstructive sleep apnea: a population health perspective. Am J Respir Crit Care Med 2002; 165(9):1217–39.

[76] Pankow W, Lies A, Lohmann FW, et al. Sleep-disordered breathing and hypertension. N Engl J Med 2000;343(13):966–7.

[77] Ali N, Davies R, Fleetham J, et al. The acute effects of continuous positive airway pressure and oxygen administration on blood pressure during obstructive sleep apnea. Chest 1992; 101(6):1526–32.

[78] Dimsdale JE, Loredo JS, Profant J. Effect of continuous positive airway pressure on blood pressure: a placebo trial. Hypertension 2000;35(1):144–7.

[79] Pepperell JC, Ramdassingh-Dow S, Crosthwaite N, et al. Ambulatory blood pressure after therapeutic and subtherapeutic nasal continuous positive airway pressure for obstructive sleep apnoea: a randomised parallel trial. Lancet 2002;359(9302): 204–10.

[80] Becker HF, Jerrentrup A, Ploch T, et al. Effect of nasal continuous positive airway pressure

treatment on blood pressure in patients with obstructive sleep apnea. Circulation 2003;107(1): 68–73.

[81] Logan AG, Perlikowski SM, Mente A, et al. High prevalence of unrecognized sleep apnoea in drug-resistant hypertension. J Hypertens 2001; 19(12):2271–7.

[82] Engleman HMGK, Martin SE, Kingshott RN, et al. Ambulatory blood pressure on and off continuous positive airway pressure therapy for the sleep apnea/hypopnea syndrome: effects in "non-dippers". Sleep 1996;19(5):378–81.

[83] Barbe F, Mayoralas LR, Duran J, et al. Treatment with continuous positive airway pressure is not effective in patients with sleep apnea but no

daytime sleepiness. a randomized, controlled trial. Ann Intern Med 2001;134(11):1015–23.

[84] Robinson GV, Smith DM, Langford BA, et al. Continuous positive airway pressure does not reduce blood pressure in nonsleepy hypertensive OSA patients. Eur Respir J 2006;27(6): 1229–35.

[85] Hui DS, To KW, Ko FW, et al. Nasal CPAP reduces systemic blood pressure in patients with obstructive sleep apnoea and mild sleepiness. Thorax 2006;61(12):1083–90.

[86] Norman D, Loredo JS, Nelesen RA, et al. Effects of continuous positive airway pressure versus supplemental oxygen on 24-hour ambulatory blood pressure. Hypertension 2006;47(5):840–5.

ELSEVIER
SAUNDERS

SLEEP
MEDICINE
CLINICS

Sleep Med Clin 2 (2007) 87–97

Sleep and Breathing in Cystic Fibrosis

Amanda J. Piper, PhD[a,b,*], Peter T.P. Bye, MBBS, PhD[c,d,e],
Ronald R. Grunstein, MD, PhD[b,c]

Cystic fibrosis (CF) is a common, autosomal recessive disorder that is associated with a defect in the protein that regulates the movement of salt and water across the epithelial cell membrane, resulting in dehydration of secretions and obstruction of lumens and ducts. Major clinical manifestations of CF include progressive lung disease, pancreatic insufficiency, and gut and biliary disease. There is usually an elevated concentration of sweat electrolytes. Abnormalities in the respiratory system arise from retention of mucus, leading to chronic infection and inflammation of the airways. With time this will create obstruction of the airways and gas trapping, altering lung mechanics and gas exchange.

Death is usually attributable to cor pulmonale and respiratory failure [1].

Since the early 1980s, a number of studies have looked at sleep and nocturnal breathing in this population. However, most have been concerned with identifying the appearance of hypoxemia during sleep and the mechanisms underlying this. There remains a paucity of data examining sleep quality and its relationship to daytime function. In particular, longitudinal studies examining the links between nocturnal gas exchange and disease progression are lacking. In this chapter, we will outline current knowledge of sleep and breathing in this population, its impact on

This work has been supported by the National Health and Medical Research Council, Australia.
[a] Respiratory Failure Service, Department of Respiratory and Sleep Medicine, Level 11, E Block, Royal Prince Alfred Hospital, Missenden Road, Camperdown, NSW 2050, Australia
[b] Sleep and Circadian Group, Woolcock Institute of Medical Research, University of Sydney, Building F, Level 6, 88 Mallett St., Camperdown, NSW, 2050, Australia
[c] Department of Respiratory and Sleep Medicine, Royal Prince Alfred Hospital, Missenden Road, Camperdown, NSW 2050, Australia
[d] Cystic Fibrosis Unit, Royal Prince Alfred Hospital, Missenden Road, Camperdown, NSW 2050, Australia
[e] Cystic Fibrosis Group, Woolcock Institute of Medical Research, University of Sydney, Building F, Level 6, 88 Mallett St, Camperdown, NSW, 2050, Australia
* Corresponding author. Respiratory Failure Service, Department of Respiratory and Sleep Medicine, Level 11, E Block, Royal Prince Alfred Hospital, Missenden Road, Camperdown, NSW 2050, Australia.
E-mail address: ajp@mail.med.usyd.edu.au (A.J. Piper).

doi:10.1016/j.jsmc.2006.11.012

daytime function, and the potential effects of intervention.

Nocturnal ventilation and gas exchange

The earliest and most frequently reported studies of sleep in CF have examined the relationship between sleep and nocturnal hypoxemia. In a study of nine patients with moderate to severe lung disease, four were found to have significant falls in SaO_2, most commonly during rapid eye movement (REM) sleep [2]. Likewise in a group of 20 young adult subjects with CF, it was observed that the largest decreases in SaO_2 occurred during REM sleep, with REM SaO_2 almost continuously lower than the level seen in non–rapid eye movement (NREM) sleep [3,4]. During the transition from NREM to REM sleep, a decrease in tonic intercostal and diaphragmatic muscle activity was observed [3]. A decrease in the baseline of both the rib cage and abdominal magnetometers when the subject changed from NREM to REM sleep was also noted, which was attributed to a decrease in functional residual capacity (FRC) [3]. From these studies the authors concluded that worsening of ventilation perfusion mismatching during sleep from a fall in FRC was largely responsible for the decrement in saturation seen during REM sleep. This would then be made worse by transient episodes of hypoventilation [3,4].

In a study of six adolescent males with moderate to severe CF lung disease, ventilation was measured during sleep to determine the effect of NREM and REM sleep on absolute levels of ventilation, breathing pattern, and inspiratory effort [5]. There was a decrease in tidal volume, minute ventilation, and mean inspiratory flow between the awake, NREM, and REM sleep states, with the greatest falls occurring during phasic REM sleep. Breathing pattern was also more variable during REM compared with either NREM or wakefulness. From these results it was speculated that hypoventilation was the most likely cause of the hypoxemia seen in REM sleep in these patients. In an elaborate study designed to better define the contribution hypoventilation and ventilation-perfusion mismatching play in sleep hypoxemia in patients with CF, five adult patients with moderate lung disease slept in a horizontal body plethysmograph with a tightly fitted facemask and an esophageal balloon [6]. Sleep-associated reductions in tidal volume and minute ventilation were again noted with the transition from wakefulness to NREM sleep. No changes in either upper airway or lower airway resistance were seen, nor were any changes in FRC between wakefulness and any NREM sleep stage recorded. However, an NREM-associated reduction in $P_{0.1}$ was observed, suggesting a reduction in respiratory

neuromuscular output. Unfortunately, probably because of the rigorous nocturnal monitoring that was undertaken, no patient was able to achieve REM sleep, where the greatest changes in ventilation and gas exchange have been shown to occur. Therefore, it remains unclear if the mechanisms underlying desaturation in NREM sleep are the same when patients move into REM sleep.

Direct measurements of ventilation were made in a group of 13 patients with moderate to severe lung disease and demonstrated a nonsignificant reduction in minute ventilation from wakefulness to NREM with a further significant fall during REM sleep, confirming the presence of hypoventilation during this sleep stage [7]. Most of the fall in minute ventilation could be accounted for by a fall in tidal volume, as has been previously reported [5,6]. While falls in minute ventilation have been a consistent finding in those studies examining this, data on respiratory rate have been less consistent. Some studies have reported a reduction from NREM to REM [8], no change from wake to sleep [5,6], or an increase from wake to both NREM and REM sleep [7].

Understanding the mechanisms underlying changes in gas exchange and breathing during sleep is important as it can influence the therapeutic interventions that are subsequently used. In contrast to many other medical conditions, the presence of frank apneic episodes, snoring, or paradoxical movement of the chest wall is unusual in this population [5,7], with the main abnormality being sleep hypoxemia with hypopneas, especially during REM sleep (Fig. 1). The current evidence suggests that while ventilation-perfusion inequality contributes to the hypoxemia seen, hypoventilation, particularly during REM sleep, is the major contributing factor to the sustained falls in saturation and rises in carbon dioxide that can occur in patients with severe lung disease [9]. Therefore, therapies addressing falls in alveolar ventilation may be more effective than simply increasing oxygenation alone [7].

Sleep quality in cystic fibrosis

Patients with CF commonly report disturbed sleep, even during periods of clinical stability [10–12]. There are many reasons why sleep may be abnormal in this population, with the most obvious being those related to the respiratory system. Alterations in lung mechanics and gas exchange can increase the work of breathing [13] and this increased effort could consequently disturb sleep [14]. Cough, secondary to accumulated secretions and airway inflammation, can prevent the patient from entering deeper stages of sleep [2,4,8]. Children with CF and their parents report cough

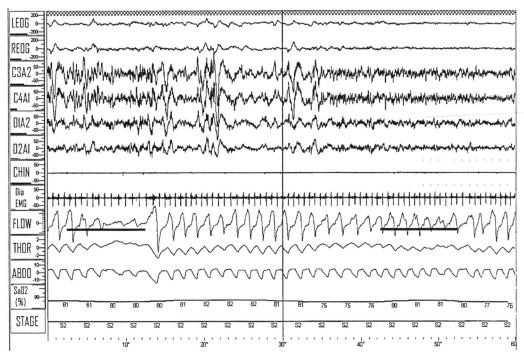

Fig. 1. Epoch of sleep from a patient with CF and severe lung disease taken just as the patient is moving from NREM sleep into REM sleep. Hypopneas (reduced flow) occurring on a background of already low baseline saturation (around 80%) results in further falls in SpO_2 (minimum 75%), despite the patient being on supplemental oxygen therapy.

disturbing their sleep more commonly than age-matched controls [12]. β-agonists to reduce bronchial obstruction and improve lung function are commonly used [15]. Although this has been shown to improve overnight oxygenation [16], it may also alter sleep quality [17]. Nasal obstruction and sinus problems could further disrupt sleep. Problems with the gastrointestinal system could be another source of sleep disruption in these patients. Symptoms of gastroesophageal reflux, heartburn, and regurgitation have been found to be more frequent in CF patients than in their siblings [18]. Symptomatic and silent reflux are common both before and after lung transplantation, and may contribute to progressive lung damage before transplantation as well as to the development of obliterative bronchiolitis in some patients after transplantation [19,20]; however, there have been no studies examining sleep quality and the presence of reflux in this population. Other CF-related gastrointestinal disorders such as nocturnal visits to the bathroom have also been reported to disturb sleep in children with CF [12].

There is only limited information regarding objectively measured sleep architecture and sleep quality in this population. In a number of the early studies, time spent in NREM and REM sleep did not differ markedly from that reported in healthy young adults [2,3]. In a study comparing sleep quality in 14 adult patients with moderate lung disease to that of 8 healthy control subjects, no significant differences in sleep efficiency, sleep architecture, or arousal frequency were found between the two groups, despite the presence of significant sleep hypoxemia in the CF group [14]. Similarly, in a group of stable CF patients with moderate to severe lung disease (mean forced expiratory volume at one second 36% predicted), sleep architecture was not different from that reported for healthy subjects [21]. In 20 CF patients with moderate lung disease studied during a period of clinical stability [22], sleep macrostructure and frequency of arousals were similar to that seen in previously reported control groups [14]. In contrast, sleep efficiency [8,17], total sleep time (TST) [17], and REM sleep [8] were significantly reduced compared with concurrently studied healthy age-matched controls. Polysomnographic variables have also been studied in 19 very young children (mean age 13 months) and compared with 20 age- and sex-matched healthy subjects [23]. No differences between sleep architecture or apnea-hypopnea index were found between the two groups. Therefore, the differences in objective sleep quality so far reported in patients with CF seem to likely be a result of the severity of lung disease, with those patients with severe pulmonary disease generally experiencing poorer sleep efficiency, less time in REM sleep, and more time awake after sleep onset [8,17]. There is also evidence that with increasing age, sleep quality worsens and sleep duration decreases [7]. Longitudinal studies examining sleep quality with progressive deterioration of lung disease would be of value in better understanding these differences.

Arousals from sleep in the face of abnormal breathing with oxygen desaturation and rises in carbon dioxide would be expected to lead to sleep disruption and fragmentation. However, a number of studies have shown that falls in oxygen saturation frequently do not result in arousals, and arousals frequently occur in the absence of changes in breathing or gas exchange [4,8]. Although some studies have reported more frequent brief awakenings during the night in patients with CF compared with healthy controls [8,17], the arousal index reported in many studies has been within the normal range [14,22]. Questionnaire data have suggested an inverse association between forced expiratory volume at one second (FEV_1) and the frequency of awakenings with nocturnal cough in children with CF [12]. This is in keeping with objective measures of sleep quality in patients with severe lung disease, which suggest that bouts of coughing can coincide with arousals, and that in patients with CF there are a greater number of sleep stage changes per hour of sleep and more awakenings longer than 5 minutes compared with controls [8]. However, there is a lack of sleep microstructure analysis or electroencephalogram (EEG) spectral analysis to confirm these findings.

Irrespective of results from monitored sleep, a significant number of patients with CF perceive their sleep to be of poor quality [10,11,17]. Because pulmonary symptoms and exacerbations are episodic in CF, one of the criticisms of using polysomnography in this population has been that a single study night may fail to reflect true sleep quality over a more prolonged time period [11]. A first night effect has been shown in these patients with reduced sleep efficiency, increased REM latency, and increased wakefulness following sleep onset compared with a subsequent night's sleep, although sleep-related hypoxemia and respiratory events were not affected [21]. Therefore, other tools to evaluate sleep quality and disturbance have been more recently used in an attempt to better monitor sleep-wake habits in these patients.

The Pittsburgh Sleep Quality Index (PSQI) is a validated questionnaire that examines seven areas of sleep including sleep quality, latency, efficiency, and disturbances. In a study comparing the PSQI to full polysomnography in 33 patients with CF,

those patients with low PSQI scores (ie, better subjective sleep quality) were shown to have significantly better sleep efficiency and a greater percentage of REM sleep than those with higher global scores [10]. The components of the PSQI that appeared to contribute most to the poor sleep perceived by CF patients were those related to sleep latency and sleep disturbance [10,11]. In addition, poorer sleep quality was associated with more severely impaired lung function and worse gas exchange [10]. Therefore, the PSQI has been suggested as a useful screening tool to identify CF patients who are at risk for sleep disturbance, especially if their FEV_1 is reduced [11]. The questionnaire is easy to administer and could be used to determine the impact of alterations in therapy or changes in physiological status.

Several studies have also examined the usefulness of actigraphy in this population [11,12]. Using wrist actigraphy, Jankelowitz and colleagues [11] measured sleep quality including sleep duration, efficiency, and fragmentation index in 20 young adult patients with a range of lung disease severity and compared this to age-matched control subjects. They found that total sleep time, sleep efficiency, and sleep latency were similar between the CF patients and control subjects. However, in the CF patients sleep was significantly more fragmented, with more night-to-night variability in the fragmentation index (FI) and immobile time (IT). There were also small but significant associations between FEV_1 and sleep disturbance. Self-perceived sleep quality was also poor. Actigraphy has also been used in children and adolescents to measure sleep quality [12]. Children with CF were found to have significantly lower sleep efficiency and more frequent awakenings from sleep compared with control subjects. FEV_1 correlated positively with sleep duration and sleep efficiency, and negatively with the duration and number of awakenings after sleep onset.

Sleep and breathing during acute exacerbations

Most studies looking at sleep and breathing in patients with CF have been performed during periods of clinical stability. However, one of the hallmarks of this disease is the frequent infective exacerbations these patients experience, associated with increased cough, sputum production, and decrements in gas exchange. However, there have been few studies exploring the effect of acute exacerbations on sleep and nocturnal gas exchange. Although pulmonary exacerbations have been found to have a profound negative impact on physical and psychosocial health-related quality of life [24], the specific elements of the exacerbation that contribute to this, including the impact on sleep quality, have not been explored. In the stable state, cough has been shown to affect sleep quality by arousing the patient from sleep [2,8]. Pulmonary exacerbations are defined by clinical criteria including an increase in cough [25,26]; however, there has been little study of cough during an exacerbation and how it could affect sleep quality. Using digital sound recordings, substantial falls in both daytime and nocturnal cough rates in adults treated for an exacerbation of CF were found [27]. In contrast, no significant improvement between admission and discharge cough counts were seen in a study of children with CF admitted with an infective exacerbation despite significant improvements in lung function [28]. However any relationship between changes in sleep quality and changes in nocturnal cough were not addressed in either study.

In addition to cough, gas exchange is also likely to worsen during an exacerbation and this could further affect sleep quality. In a study of 45 children admitted for acute exacerbations of CF, 38 were found to have evidence of clinically significant sleep-related desaturation (defined as a saturation of 4% or more below their stable clinic value for more than 5 minutes) on their first admission night [29]. Although the time spent desaturated during sleep improved markedly with therapy over a 10-day period, falling from 122 (152) minutes to 21 (31) minutes, 34 patients continued to desaturate nocturnally after treatment. Villa and colleagues [23] studied 19 CF infants (mean age 13 months) with normal lung function with full polysomnography. When studied, seven children had symptoms compatible with mild respiratory tract inflammation, and each of these children experienced oxygen desaturation during sleep that was not seen in the asymptomatic CF group or the controls. These authors concluded that even during episodes of mild airway inflammation, infants with CF may experience oxygen desaturation during sleep.

Pond and Conway [30] analyzed lung function and SaO_2 during 147 episodes of exacerbation in 47 patients with CF looking for predictors of nocturnal desaturation during these episodes. As in previous studies [31,32], only a modest correlation between lung function and nocturnal saturation was found. They concluded that spirometric parameters could not be used to predict the presence of nocturnal desaturation during pulmonary exacerbations and that nocturnal oximetry was needed to identify those patients experiencing desaturation during sleep.

In a study of 22 patients during an acute exacerbation, sleep quality and arterial blood gases were compared with another group of CF patients who underwent the same testing procedures during a period of clinical stability [22]. Pulmonary exacerbations were not only associated with poorer sleep quality but also impaired daytime function compared with periods of clinical stability. Sleep efficiency was reduced along with time spent in REM sleep while an increase in time awake after sleep onset was also seen.

Impact of sleep on daytime function

How sleep quality and nocturnal gas exchange affect daytime function has received limited attention in this population. Although patients with CF report significant sleep disturbance [10–12], daytime sleepiness as measured subjectively by Epworth Sleepiness Scale (ESS) [11,17] or objectively by multiple sleep latency testing [17] is not different from that seen in age-matched controls. However, one study found patients with severe stable disease had significantly lower levels of activation and happiness while levels of fatigue were greater compared with controls [17]. These changes in daytime functioning correlated with parameters of sleep quality but did not correlate with daytime or nocturnal hypoxemia.

Episodes of pulmonary exacerbation have been shown to adversely affect sleep quality as well as daytime performance of tasks assessing reaction time, concentration, and concrete reasoning [22]. By the end of a 10- to 14-day treatment period, significant improvements in objective sleep quality and nocturnal hypoxia occurred, along with improved neurocognitive performance and subjective reports of sleepiness, exhaustion, and activation. These results suggest it is possible to reverse some of the impairment caused by sleep disruption and/or hypoxemia in these patients, although further work is needed to determine which therapies are most likely to achieve these outcomes.

In patients with severe stable disease, deficits in objective neurocognitive functioning have been reported, with CF patients performing at around 60% of that seen in the control group [17]. Further, performance of these tasks did not improve over the day as was seen in the control subjects. Unlike patients with chronic obstructive pulmonary disease (COPD), neither daytime nor nocturnal oxygenation were found to be related to this impairment of performance, and there was no clear relationship between changes in objective sleep quality and daytime performance. However, the impairment of performance was internally consistent with the patients' subjective reports of fatigue and activation. It was suggested that in these young adults, neurocognitive function may be less sensitive to hypoxemia compared with older COPD patients [17] and this may explain, at least in part, why intervention with long-term nocturnal oxygen therapy has not been shown to result in improvements in neuro-cognitive performance [33]. It has been proposed that the deficits seen in patients with CF may be related to chronic sleep deprivation [17], which would be consistent with the patients' subjective reports of sleep disturbance. Considerably more work needs to be done in this area to improve our understanding of the consequences of sleep quality on daytime functioning and the impact of therapies on this.

Sleep breathing abnormalities and disease progression

Investigations to date regarding sleep and cystic fibrosis have primarily focused on the impact of the hypoxic insult patients may experience, and the role this could play in the development of pulmonary hypertension. However, the impact that sleep hypoxemia and disruption may have on other systems has not been widely addressed.

Repeated chest infections are a classic characteristic of patients with CF lung disease, with *Pseudomonas aeruginosa* being the most common pathogen. Under conditions of hypoxia this pathogen changes phenotype [34], promoting resistance to secondary host mechanisms [35], which could contribute to further chronic lung damage [36]. It has also been speculated that hypoxia could up-regulate lung inflammation in CF by activating transcription factors such as nuclear factor κB (NFκB). This would increase the expression of cytokines, which in turn would attract neutrophils, initiating and promoting airway inflammation and lung damage [36]. However, whether oxygen therapy is effective in down-regulating this inflammatory cascade is uncertain especially as inflammation occurs from early on in the disease course. In addition, hypoxic gradients have been demonstrated, localized deep in airway mucus plugs where bacteria may be relatively inaccessible. In healthy individuals, the immune response is adversely affected by sleep loss [37], and impaired sleep has been implicated in increased risk of infection in some populations [38]. It is possible that in a disorder such as CF that is characterized by chronic infection and inflammation, sleep loss, or fragmentation could further worsen host defenses to infection resulting in delayed recovery or a more rapid progression of lung disease.

Many patients with CF also develop diabetes [39], and this is associated with a deterioration in pulmonary function and increased mortality [40]. In healthy subjects, sleep loss has been associated with decreased insulin sensitivity [41]. In patients with obstructive sleep apnea (OSA), the extent of insulin resistance has been shown to be related to the severity of the hypoxic stress [42]. Theoretically, sleep disturbance in CF could add to the existing susceptibility to glucose intolerance seen in this population. Given the evidence in other medical disorders of the adverse consequences of sleep loss and fragmentation on a number of aspects of immune and metabolic function, further investigation in patients with CF would appear warranted.

Identifying and monitoring sleep and gas exchange

Considering the impact abnormal sleep breathing could have on disease progression and daytime function, early identification of at-risk patients in whom further monitoring and intervention is required would appear to be an important therapeutic strategy. To this end, a number of investigators have attempted to identify the presence and severity of sleep hypoxemia using daytime assessments of clinical status and pulmonary function. Because both exercise and sleep are potential stressors of the respiratory system, several studies have examined the relationship between these states and oxygenation [14,43,44]. Although there is a general association, exercise parameters do not add to the ability to predict patients likely to desaturate during sleep [44]. Nonhypoxemic patients with CF have been shown to desaturate more during sleep than during exercise [14,43], although the magnitude of desaturation during sleep cannot be predicted from either their awake SpO_2 or the magnitude of exercise-related desaturation [43]. More simple parameters such as resting awake SpO_2 and FEV_1 have been studied to determine their ability to identify patients likely to be at risk of desaturation during sleep. As might be expected, those patients with more severe disease and lower awake resting SpO_2 spend more of their sleep time at SpO_2 levels below 90% [31,44,45]. Montgomery and colleagues [32] found that patients with a resting PaO_2 higher than 70 mm Hg ($SpO_2 > 92\%$) spent less than 20% of their sleep time with SpO_2 below 90%. In contrast, those patients with a resting PaO_2 less than 60 mmHg ($SpO_2 < 91\%$) spent more than 80% of their sleep time below 90%. Versteegh and colleagues [31] reported that an awake resting SpO_2 of 94% was the most discriminatory measurement for predicting sleep-related desaturation in CF, with a 50% likelihood of nocturnal desaturation being present below this value. Although sleep-related desaturation occurred only in those subjects with an FEV_1 less than 65%, the addition of spirometric variables did not add significantly to the discriminatory power of SpO_2 alone. Other authors have likewise reported an awake SpO_2 below 94% as indicative of a patient with CF being at risk of nocturnal desaturation, but not its severity [45,46]. In a stepwise discriminant analysis, percent predicted FEV_1 and resting SpO_2 were identified as parameters that could best identify patients unlikely to experience nocturnal desaturation [44]; however, the equation could only predict 26% of cases that were likely to desaturate during sleep. These results highlight the limited utility of non-sleep measurements in identifying patients with nocturnal desaturation, and the importance of using nocturnal oximetry in patients to detect early changes in nocturnal gas exchange.

Intervention for sleep-disordered breathing and gas exchange

Identifying and treating sleep hypoxemia has been considered an important therapeutic goal in the management of patients with CF because of the contribution this phenomenon plays in the development and progression of pulmonary hypertension and cor pulmonale. A significant proportion of patients with CF develop subclinical pulmonary hypertension and this appears to be strongly associated with hypoxemia, independent of pulmonary function [47]. Since cor pulmonale is a poor prognostic sign [48], correcting hypoxemia and lowering elevated pulmonary artery pressure is considered an important aspect of disease management.

Work by Goldring and colleagues [49] established the role hypoxia played in the pathogenesis of pulmonary hypertension and its potential reversibility in CF. Even in those with mild pulmonary hypertension, short-term oxygen administration has been shown to decrease pulmonary pressure and resistance while increasing systemic vascular resistance [50]. However, once moderate to severe pulmonary hypertension develops, use of oxygen therapy may only be partially effective in returning pressures to normal levels [49]. Therefore, relieving pulmonary vasoconstriction before irreversible vascular damage has developed is seen to be of crucial importance. Since nocturnal hypoxemia can occur before the development of awake changes in blood gases, identifying patients who are exhibiting nocturnal desaturation and intervening early could slow down disease progression. Although the threshold of nocturnal desaturation that is physiologically significant has not been identified, a recent consensus report on CF adult care recommended that nocturnal oxygen should be used if oxygen saturation was less than 88% to 90% for 10% or more of total sleep time [51]. However, there is currently no evidence to demonstrate that such intervention has any impact on the progression of pulmonary hypertension or survival. Data are also limited regarding the impact of improved nocturnal gas exchange on daytime function and quality of life.

Several studies have examined the use of short-term nocturnal oxygen therapy on sleep and breathing [7,8,52], using a single-night crossover design. The acute effects of nocturnal low flow oxygen on sleep quality, sleep disordered breathing, and nocturnal gas exchange was studied in 10 patients with severe stable CF lung disease [8]. The progressive fall in SpO_2 from wakefulness to NREM and REM sleep that occurred during the control night breathing room air was almost eliminated with the use of oxygen therapy. However, this had no impact on sleep quality, with sleep efficiency, sleep stage distribution, and awakenings longer than 5 minutes per hour of sleep time being no different from that seen during the room air night. Likewise, oxygen therapy did not attenuate the fall in minute ventilation from slow wave to REM sleep. Transcutaneous carbon dioxide ($TcCO_2$) levels reached their highest values in each sleep state during oxygen breathing compared with room air, with the overall greatest rises recorded during REM sleep. The average maximal rise was 5.6 mm Hg while breathing room air and this increased a further 5 mm Hg with low-flow oxygen, which the authors felt was clinically unimportant.

Two later studies involving 19 patients with moderate to severe lung disease have examined the effects of oxygen on sleep and ventilation [7,52]. Significant improvements in nocturnal SpO_2 were achieved with the administration of supplemental oxygen in both studies, although rises in $TcCO_2$ were also noted during oxygen administration, with two patients reporting morning headache [52]. Oxygen therapy had no impact on the fall in minute ventilation or tidal volume that occurred from the awake state to NREM and REM sleep [7]. In neither study was sleep quality modified significantly by oxygen therapy, with no change in total sleep time, sleep latency, or arousals. Milross and colleagues [7] also found no change in sleep architecture with oxygen therapy, in contrast to Gozal [52] who reported a significant increase in the amount of REM sleep from 12% to 18% of total sleep time [52]. Since the above three studies used oxygen for a single night only in a sleep laboratory, no data regarding the patient's perception of sleep quality or impact on daytime functioning were measured.

Only one study has investigated the longer-term effects of nocturnal oxygen therapy on disease progression and psychosocial function in patients with CF [33]. In a randomized, double-blind study of 28 patients with severe lung disease (mean FEV_1 34%-38% predicted), either nocturnal humidified oxygen or room air was commenced with follow-up over a 26-month period. Patients randomized to oxygen used this for an average of 7 hours per night compared with 5.3 hours per night for the air group. Disease progression was monitored by nutritional status, pulmonary function, exercise ability, right ventricular ejection fraction, and blood gases. At 12 months, there was no difference in any of these measurements between the two groups. Mortality rate and frequency of hospitalizations also did not differ. Standardized tests assessing mood, self-esteem, and cognitive function were within normal limits at baseline and demonstrated no significant change over the first year of follow-up. The only difference noted was an increased likelihood of those assigned to oxygen therapy continuing to attend school or work on a daily basis compared with the air group who decreased their participation in such activities substantially over the study period. However, there were a number of limitations to this study, including the small number of patients and the relatively short daily use of oxygen. In the two long-term oxygen trials in COPD, the longer the patients used oxygen in the 24-hour period, the greater the improvement in mortality [53,54]. In the CF trial, the daily duration of oxygen use may have been

inadequate to obtain a significant benefit [33]. On the other hand, differences in pulmonary pathophysiology between the two conditions may mean that CF patients show less therapeutic responsiveness to oxygen therapy [33,55].

Given that the main contributory factor to hypoxemia during sleep in CF is the drop in minute ventilation going from wakefulness to REM sleep [5,7], interest in nocturnal noninvasive ventilatory support (NIV) has arisen. While the technique has been used widely in CF patients with acute on chronic respiratory failure [56–58], as with oxygen therapy, there is little evidence to guide when and how this therapy should be used. Gozal [52] demonstrated that NIV in the form of bi-level ventilatory support was as effective as supplemental oxygen in improving SpO$_2$ during sleep in patients with moderate to severe lung disease. In contrast to supplemental oxygen, improvements in sleep SpO$_2$ were achieved without inducing significant rises in carbon dioxide. Improved sleep breathing occurred without adversely affecting sleep architecture or inducing more frequent arousals from sleep. However,

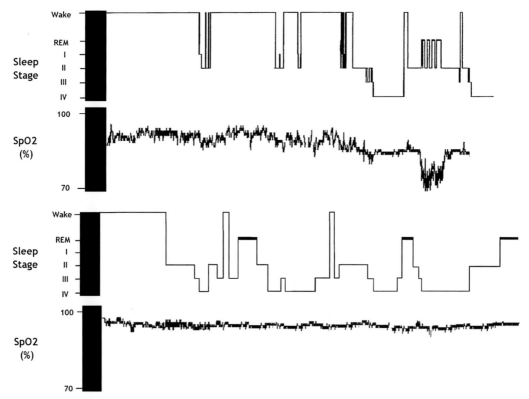

Fig. 2. Top panel illustrates poor-quality sleep, with long periods of wakefulness during the night. When the patient did sleep, baseline SpO$_2$ was low and fell further during the single period of disrupted REM sleep that was achieved. The patient was using nocturnal oxygen during this study. In the *bottom panel* the patient has been placed on NIV with supplemental oxygen. Nocturnal saturation improved along with sleep architecture.

two of the eight patients enrolled in the study withdrew because of intolerance to the mask or pressure, and of the remaining six patients, four stated a preference for low-flow oxygen rather than NIV. It has also been shown that the REM-related hypoventilation that normally occurs with room air and low flow oxygen therapy can be ameliorated with NIV by maintaining minute ventilation, thereby preventing oxyhemoglobin desaturation (   ) [7]. As has been shown previously [52], NIV prevents the rise in $TcCO_2$ that occurs during room air and low flow oxygen breathing, with improvements in pH and lower morning CO_2 values after a night of NIV compared with low flow oxygen [7]. Although it has been suggested that use of NIV may delay the onset of awake hypoxemia and hypercapnia by preventing sleep hypoventilation, longer-term data to support this are lacking. Recent preliminary data from a 6-week, randomized crossover trial comparing NIV to oxygen and air has provided some evidence that NIV can improve quality of life, nocturnal hypoventilation, and exercise capacity in hypercapnic CF patients. However, no changes in lung function, sleep architecture, or daytime hypercapnia were seen [59]. Further studies confirming such findings are needed.

Summary

Current evidence suggests that sleep disturbance is common in CF patients, and that chronic sleep loss may have a definite impact on psychosocial and neurocognitive functioning. Nocturnal gas exchange worsens as lung disease progresses, with adverse clinical consequences, not only the development of pulmonary hypertension, but also potentially for metabolic and immune function. Further studies are required to identify strategies that can improve sleep quality and gas exchange in these patients, and to determine if such interventions have an impact on quality of life and survival.

References

[1] Davis PB. Cystic fibrosis since 1938. Am J Respir Crit Care Med 2006;173(5):475–82.

[2] Stokes DC, McBride JT, Wall MA, et al. Sleep hypoxemia in young adults with cystic fibrosis. Am J Dis Child 1980;134(8):741–3.

[3] Muller NL, Francis PW, Gurwitz D, et al. Mechanism of hemoglobin desaturation during rapid-eye-movement sleep in normal subjects and in patients with cystic fibrosis. Am Rev Respir Dis 1980;121(3):463–9.

[4] Francis PW, Muller NL, Gurwitz D, et al. Hemoglobin desaturation: its occurrence during sleep in patients with cystic fibrosis. Am J Dis Child 1980;134(8):734–40.

[5] Tepper RS, Skatrud JB, Dempsey JA. Ventilation and oxygenation changes during sleep in cystic fibrosis. Chest 1983;84(4):388–93.

[6] Ballard Rd, Sutarik JM, Clover CW, et al. Effects of non-REM sleep on ventilation and respiratory mechanics in adults with cystic fibrosis. Am J Respir Crit Care Med 1996;153(1):266–71.

[7] Milross MA, Piper AJ, Norman M, et al. Low flow oxygen and bilevel ventilatory support: effects on ventilation during sleep in cystic fibrosis. Am J Respir Crit Care Med 2001;163(1):129–34.

[8] Spier S, Rivlin J, Hughes D, et al. The effect of oxygen on sleep, blood gases, and ventilation in cystic fibrosis. Am Rev Respir Dis 1984;129(5):712–8.

[9] Piper AJ, Milross MM, Bye PTP. Sleep and breathing in cystic fibrosis. Sleep: A comprehensive handbook. In: Lee-Chiong T, editor. Hoboken (NJ): John Wiley & Sons, Inc.; 2006. p. 685–92

[10] Milross MA, Piper AJ, Normal M, et al. Subjective sleep quality in cystic fibrosis. Sleep Medicine 2002;3:205–12.

[11] Jankelowitz L, Reid KJ, Wolfe L, et al. Cystic fibrosis patients have poor sleep quality despite normal sleep latency and efficiency. Chest 2005;127(5):1593–9.

[12] Amin R, Bean J, Burklow K, et al. The relationship between sleep disturbance and pulmonary function in stable pediatric cystic fibrosis patients. Chest 2005;128(3):1357–63.

[13] Hart N, Polkey MI, Clement A, et al. Changes in pulmonary mechanics with increasing disease severity in children and young adults with cystic fibrosis. Am J Respir Crit Care Med 2002;166(1):61–6.

[14] Bradley S, Solin P, Wilson J, et al. Hypoxemia and hypercapnia during exercise and sleep in patients with cystic fibrosis. Chest 1999;116(3):647–54.

[15] Konig P, Gayer D, Barbero GJ, et al. Short-term and long-term effects of albuterol aerosol therapy in cystic fibrosis: a preliminary report. Pediatr Pulmonol 1995;20(4):205–14.

[16] Salvatore D, D'Andria M. Effects of salmeterol on arterial oxyhemoglobin saturations in patients with cystic fibrosis. Pediatr Pulmonol 2002;34(1):11–5.

[17] Dancey DR, Tullis ED, Heslegrave R, et al. Sleep quality and daytime function in adults with cystic fibrosis and severe lung disease. Eur Respir J 2002;19(3):504–10.

[18] Scott RB, O'Loughlin EV, Gall DG. Gastroesophageal reflux in patients with cystic fibrosis. J Pediatr 1985;106(2):223–7.

[19] Reid KL, McKenzie FN, Menkis AH, et al. Importance of chronic aspiration in recipients of heart-lung transplants. Lancet 1990;333(8709):206–8.

[20] Button BM, Roberts S, Kotsimbos C, et al. Gastroesophageal reflux (symptomatic and silent): a potentially significant problem in patients

with cystic fibrosis before and after lung transplantation. J Heart Lung Transplant 2005;24(10):1522–9.

[21] Milross MA, Piper AJ, Norman M, et al. Night-to-night variability in sleep in cystic fibrosis. Sleep Med 2002;3(3):213–9.

[22] Dobbin CJ, Bartlett D, Melehan K, et al. The effect of infective exacerbations on sleep and neurobehavioral function in cystic fibrosis. Am J Respir Crit Care Med 2005;172(1):99–104.

[23] Villa MP, Pagani J, Lucidi V, et al. Nocturnal oximetry in infants with cystic fibrosis. Arch Dis Child 2001;84(1):50–4.

[24] Britto MT, Kotagal UR, Hornung RW, et al. Impact of recent pulmonary exacerbations on quality of life in patients with cystic fibrosis. Chest 2002;121(1):64–72.

[25] Fuchs HJ, Borowitz DS, Christiansen DH, et al. Effect of aerosolized recombinant human DNase on exacerbations of respiratory symptoms and on pulmonary function in patients with cystic fibrosis. The Pulmozyme Study Group. N Engl J Med 1994;331(10):637–42.

[26] Cystic Fibrosis Foundation. Microbiology and infectious disease in cystic fibrosis. Bethesda (MD): Cystic Fibrosis Foundation; 1994. p. 1–26.

[27] Smith JA, Owen EC, Jones AM, et al. Objective measurement of cough during pulmonary exerbations in adults with cystic fibrosis. Thorax 2006;61(5):425–9.

[28] Hamutcu R, Francis J, Karakoc F, et al. Objective monitoring of cough in children with cystic fibrosis. Pediatr Pulmonol 2002;34(5):331–5.

[29] Allen MB, Mellon AF, Simmonds EJ, et al. Changes in nocturnal oximetry after treatment of exacerbations in cystic fibrosis. Arch Dis Child 1993;69(2):197–201.

[30] Pond MN, Conway SP. Nocturnal oxygen desaturation and spirometric parameters in adults with cystic fibrosis. Thorax 1995;50(5):539–42.

[31] Versteegh FGA, Bogaard JM, Raatgever JW, et al. Relationship between airway obstruction, desaturation during exercise and nocturnal hypoxaemia in cystic fibrosis patients. Eur Respir J 1990;3(1):68–73.

[32] Montgomery M, Wiebicke W, Bibi H, et al. Home measurement of oxygen saturation during sleep in patients with cystic fibrosis. Pediatr Pulmonol 1989;7(1):29–34.

[33] Zinman R, Corey M, Coates AL, et al. Nocturnal home oxygen in the treatment of hypoxemic cystic fibrosis patients. J Pediatr 1989;114(3):368–77.

[34] Worlitzsch D, Tarran R, Ulrich M, et al. Effect of reduced mucus oxygen concentration in airway Pseudomonas infections of cystic fibrosis patients. J Clin Invest 2002;109(3):317–25.

[35] Donaldson SH, Boucher RC. Update on pathogenesis of cystic fibrosis lung disease. Curr Opin Pulm Med 2003;9(6):486–91.

[36] Urquhart DS, Montgomery H, Jaffe A. Assessment of hypoxia in children with cystic fibrosis. Arch Dis Child 2005;90(11):1138–43.

[37] Lange T, Perras B, Fehm HL, et al. Sleep enhances the human antibody response to hepatitis A vaccination. Psychosom Med 2003;65(5):831–5.

[38] Irwin M. Effects of sleep and sleep loss on immunity and cytokines. Brain Behav Immun 2002;16(5):503–12.

[39] Moran A, Hardin D, Rodman D, et al. Diagnosis, screening and management of cystic fibrosis related diabetes mellitus: a consensus report. Diabetes Res Clin Pract 1999;45(1):61–73.

[40] Lanng S, Thorsteinsson B, Nerup J, et al. Influence of the development of diabetes mellitus on clinical status in patients with cystic fibrosis. Eur J Pediatr 1992;151(9):684–7.

[41] Spiegel K, Leproult R, Van Cauter E. Impact of sleep debt on metabolic and endocrine function. Lancet 1999;354(9188):1435–9.

[42] Ip MS, Lam B, Ng MM, et al. Obstructive sleep apnea is independently associated with insulin resistance. Am J Respir Crit Care Med 2002;165(5):670–6.

[43] Coffey MJ, FitzGerald MX, McNicholas WT. Comparison of oxygen desaturation during sleep and exercise in patients with cystic fibrosis. Chest 1991;100(3):659–62.

[44] Frangolias DD, Wilcox PG. Predictability of oxygen desaturation during sleep in patients with cystic fibrosis. Chest 2001;119(2):434–41.

[45] Braggion C, Pradal U, Mastella G. Hemoglobin desaturation during sleep and daytime in patients with cystic fibrosis and severe airway obstruction. Acta Paediatr 1992;81(12):1002–6.

[46] Smith DL, Freeman W, Cayton RM, et al. Nocturnal hypoxaemia in cystic fibrosis: relationship to pulmonary function tests. Respir Med 1994;88(7):537–9.

[47] Fraser KL, Tullis DE, Sasson Z, et al. Pulmonary hypertension and cardiac function in adult cystic fibrosis. Chest 1999;115(5):1321–8.

[48] Stern RC, Borkat G, Hirschfeld SS, et al. Heart failure in cystic fibrosis. Treatment and prognosis of cor pulmonale with failure of the right side of the heart. Am J Dis Child 1980;134(3):267–72.

[49] Goldring RM, Fishman AP, Turino GM, et al. Pulmonary hypertension and cor pulmonale in cystic fibrosis of the pancreas. J Pediatr 1964;65(4):501–24.

[50] Davidson A, Bossuyt A, Dab I. Acute effects of oxygen, nifedipine, and diltiazem in patients with cystic fibrosis and mild pulmonary hypertension. Pediatr Pulmonol 1989;6(1):53–9.

[51] Yanakous JR, Marshall BC, Sufian B, et al. Cystic fibrosis adult care. Consensus Conference Report. Chest 2004;125:1S–39S.

[52] Gozal D. Nocturnal ventilatory support in patients with cystic fibrosis: comparison with

supplemental oxygen. Eur Respir J 1997;10(9): 1999–2003.

[53] Nocturnal Oxygen Therapy Trial Group. Continuous or nocturnal oxygen therapy in hypoxemic chronic obstructive lung disease: a clinical trial. Ann Intern Med 1980;93(3):391–8.

[54] Medical Research Council Working Party. Long-term domiciliary oxygen therapy in chronic hypoxic cor pulmonale complicating chronic bronchitis and emphysema. Lancet 1981;1(8222):681–6.

[55] Mallory GB, Fullmer JJ, Vaughan DJ. Oxygen therapy for cystic fibrosis. Cochrane Database Syst Rev 2005;4:CD003884.

[56] Hodson ME, Madden BP, Steven MH, et al. Non-invasive mechanical ventilation for cystic fibrosis patients: a potential bridge to transplantation. Eur Respir J 1991;4(5):524–7.

[57] Piper AJ, Parker S, Torzillo PJ, et al. Nocturnal nasal IPPV stabilizes patients with cystic fibrosis and hypercapnic respiratory failure. Chest 1992; 102(3):846–50.

[58] Madden BP, Kariyawasam H, Siddiqi AJ, et al. Noninvasive ventilation in cystic fibrosis patients with acute or chronic respiratory failure. Eur Respir J 2002;19(2):310–3.

[59] Young AC, Wilson JW, Kotsimbos TC, et al. Randomized placebo-controlled trial of non-invasive ventilation for hypercapnia in cystic fibrosis [abstract]. Sleep and Biological Rhythms 2006;4(Suppl 1):A9.

SLEEP
MEDICINE
CLINICS

Sleep Med Clin 2 (2007) 99–104

Sleep and Pulmonary Hypertension

Vidya Krishnan, MD, Nancy A. Collop, MD*

- The intersection of SRBDs and PH
- Mechanisms of SRBD resulting in PH
  Hypoxemia
  Hypercoagulability
  Systemic inflammation
  Other
- The effect of treatment of SRBD on PH
- PH syndromes associated
  with sleep-disordered
  breathing
  Congestive heart failure and SDB
  PPH and SDB
- Summary
- References

Pulmonary hypertension (PH) is a chronic cardiopulmonary disorder defined by elevated pulmonary arterial pressures, resulting in decreased quality of life and reduced life expectancy. Mean pulmonary arterial pressures consistent with PH are at least 25 mm Hg at rest or 30 mm Hg with exercise. The current classification of PH uses clinical criteria to distinguish between the five categories of PH ( ). The effect of sleep and its disorders on PH is not well studied. Sleep-disordered breathing may be implicated in the elevation of pulmonary arterial pressures; however, a search of the medical literature failed to find any research evaluating the relationship between PH and sleep disorders, such as insomnia, circadian rhythm disorders, restless legs syndrome or sleep-related movement disorders, hypersomnias, or parasomnias. Therefore, this review will focus on the association between sleep-related breathing disorders and pulmonary hemodynamics.

Sleep-related breathing disorders (SRBDs) are a heterogeneous cluster of diagnoses related by the common element of abnormal ventilation during sleep. Obstructive sleep apnea, central sleep apnea, and sleep-related (nocturnal) hypoventilation (SRH) are all clinical entities associated with PH. Obstructive sleep apnea is typified by recurrent complete or partial upper airway obstruction with increasingly negative intrathoracic pressure swings during inspiration, often resulting in intermittent hypoxia, hypercapnia, and recurrent arousals or awakenings. Central sleep apnea is a sleep disorder characterized by apneas and hypopneas attributable to decreased or absent respiratory drive, also resulting in intermittent hypoxia and recurrent arousals or awakenings. SRH/hypoxemia is usually associated with primary pulmonary disorders. There is no consensus on what defines this entity. Some of the definitions used are presented in .

The association between PH and SRBDs is complex. SRBDs have long been identified as a cause of PH, likely related to the intermittent hypoxia and systemic inflammatory cascade. Conversely, there is evidence that other forms of PH, particularly pulmonary arterial hypertension, are potential causes of SRBDs, reasons for which are yet to be elucidated.

The intersection of SRBDs and PH

Investigations of the effect of SRBDs on pulmonary hemodynamics have been difficult to interpret

Division of Pulmonary and Critical Care Medicine, Johns Hopkins University, 1830 East Monument Street, Room 555, Baltimore, MD 21205, USA
* Corresponding author.
E-mail address: ncollop@jhmi.edu (N.A. Collop).

because of limitations in these studies. Chronic obstructive pulmonary disease and obesity are strong and common confounding conditions that are often not adequately accounted for. Another source of ambiguity in these studies is the measurement of pulmonary arterial pressure. Whereas right heart catheterization is the gold standard measurement of PH, other studies, such as transthoracic echocardiography, are often used to evaluate right heart pressures in research studies because of their noninvasive nature. The diagnostic accuracy of transthoracic echocardiography in estimating pulmonary artery pressures is poor, especially with increasing severity of the pressure levels [1]. Studies that use transthoracic echocardiography to define patients with PH may therefore result in misclassification. Moreover, studies may use different criteria to define PH such as mean pulmonary artery pressure higher than 25 mm Hg or a systolic pulmonary artery pressure higher than 30 mm Hg. Another limitation of these studies is the use of different inclusion criteria. PH is subclassified into five categories based on clinical criteria, as outlined in Box 1. Some studies may include all forms of PH, whereas others restrict analyses to a single type of PH. The results of these studies, therefore, may not be truly comparable.

Despite these limitations, there are data to support that SRBDs can cause PH. PH is common among patients with severe obstructive sleep apnea, although *severe* PH is uncommon unless accompanied by other chronic cardiopulmonary disorders. Plausible mechanisms for development of PH

include intermittent hypoxic vasoconstriction, systemic inflammation, and hypercoagulable state. Treatment of SRBDs has been shown in small studies to improve pulmonary hemodynamics.

Studies of the prevalence of PH among patients with SRBDs (and vice versa) have been plagued by the shortcomings mentioned above. Estimates of the prevalence of PH of all types among patients with sleep apnea range from 16% to 53%, with most reporting a prevalence of approximately 20% [2–7]. In one study that sought to study the prevalence of PH among patients with obstructive sleep apnea without evidence of primary pulmonary disorder, 12 (27%) of 44 patients were found to have PH as determined by right heart catheterization [8]. In general, it is thought that patients with obstructive sleep apnea alone and PH tend to have mild PH, with an average mean pulmonary arterial pressure of less than 30 mm Hg, and tend to be older, heavier, and have worse lung function compared with patients with obstructive sleep apnea without PH [9]. Interestingly, no correlation was found in these studies between the severity of PH and the severity of the sleep-disordered breathing (as defined by the apnea-hypopnea index).

Only a single study has explored the prevalence of SRBDs among patients with pulmonary arterial hypertension. In 13 patients with severe idiopathic PH (formerly called primary PH), 10 (77%) of 13 patients displayed nocturnal hypoventilation, with more than 10% of their total sleep time spent with an oxyhemoglobin saturation less than 90%, with overt sleep apneas and hypopneas in this set of subjects noted to be rare (1.04 ± 1.93 events per hour) [10].

Mechanisms of SRBD resulting in PH

SRBDs have long been identified as a cause of PH (Fig. 1). Respiratory and metabolic derangements associated with SRBDs may cause alterations in pulmonary circulation.

Hypoxemia

An excellent review of the effects of hypoxia on PH was published by Zielinski in 2005 [11]. Whereas the systemic circulation reacts to hypoxia with vasodilation, the pulmonary vasculature reacts to hypoxia with vasoconstriction, to maintain matched ventilation and perfusion. Sustained hypoxia can result in persistent pulmonary vasoconstriction during the night. The pulmonary vasoconstrictive response to hypoxia can vary significantly between individuals, with an increase in mean pulmonary arterial pressure between 2 and 15 mm Hg [12]. Two mechanisms are postulated for pulmonary

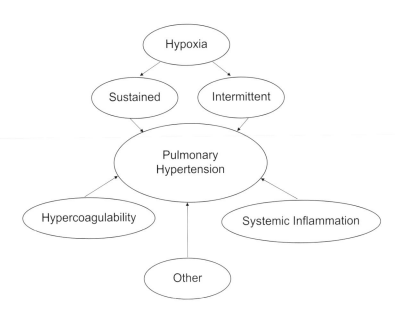

Fig. 1. Factors associated with SRBDs contributing to development of PH.

hypoxic vasoconstriction. First, oxygen-sensitive voltage-dependent potassium channels in the vascular smooth muscles are activated, resulting in membrane depolarization and subsequent vasoconstriction [13,14]. Second, there may be alterations in endothelium-mediated relaxation of pulmonary arteries [15]. Over time, the sustained hypoxia can result in remodeling of the pulmonary vasculature, with intimal smooth muscle thickening, endothelial proliferation, and fibroelastosis, resulting in diurnal PH [16–19].

In sleep apnea syndromes, the fall in oxyhemoglobin saturation with each apnea or hypopnea is determined by the preevent gas exchange, the event length, and type [20]. In severe sleep apnea, an average disordered breathing event may last 30 to 60 seconds, and may occur 500 times a night. With repetitive respiratory events throughout the night, recurrent intermittent hypoxia will ensue. Intermittent hypoxia can result in vascular oxidative stress by recurrent reoxygenation and reperfusion. Each hypoxic event can result in polymorphonuclear neutrophil activation, which results in endothelial adherence and release of free oxygen radicals [21]. Additionally, intermittent hypoxia can trigger release of potent vasoactive substances (eg, endothelin) [22], substances causing endothelial dysfunction (eg, serum soluble cell adhesion molecule-1) [23], and nitric oxide suppression [24]. The effect of these repetitive nocturnal events on persistent PH has been studied in animal models. When rats were exposed to 30 seconds of severe hypoxia followed by 30 seconds of normoxia for 8 hours a day for 5 weeks, their mean pulmonary arterial pressure increased from 20.7 ± 6.8 to 31.3 ± 7.2 mm Hg ($P < .01$) and right ventricular mass

index increased from 0.25 to 0.31 ($P < .05$) [25]. In humans, the interpretation of studies of the pathogenesis of stable PH in obstructive sleep apnea (OSA) is less consistent.

Hypercoagulability

Hypercoagulability can predispose to chronic thromboembolic disease, and subsequent PH. Obstructive sleep apnea is associated with a hypercoagulable state, measured by elevated thrombin/antithrombin III complex, fibrin, D-dimer, and von Willebrand factor antigen [26]. Other findings in patients with OSA that predict a prothrombotic state include increased platelet aggregation [27], increased blood viscosity [28], increased hematocrit [29], and increased fibrinogen levels [30]. These alterations may be mediated by an elevation in circulating levels of catecholamines [31]. It has been shown that most of these abnormalities in OSA patients can be corrected by continuous positive airway pressure (CPAP) therapy [27,30]. Whether or how much this hypercoagulable state contributes to the development of PH in patients with OSA is unknown.

Systemic inflammation

Systemic inflammation triggered by OSA has been implicated in the pathogenesis of cardiovascular complications. These same mechanisms may affect the pulmonary circulation resulting in PH. Hypoxemia and sleep deprivation can result in increased interleukin-6 (IL-6), tumor necrosis factor-alpha (TNF-alpha), and C-reactive protein (CRP), and may play a role in endothelial dysfunction [32–35].

Other

There are likely other pathophysiologic mechanisms that relate sleep-disordered breathing (SDB) to PH. OSA is associated with left ventricular dysfunction and congestive heart failure [36], which can result in elevated right heart pressures with time. Also, as mentioned earlier, OSA is associated with elevated circulating catecholamine levels [31,37], and how this may effect the pulmonary circulation is unknown and requires further study.

The effect of treatment of SRBD on PH

The impact of treatment of SRBDs on pulmonary hemodynamics has been studied in a number of small studies. Treatment of OSA with CPAP has been shown to reduce pulmonary arterial pressures in patients with and without PH. Most recently, Arias and colleagues [38] studied pulmonary hemodynamics and OSA in 23 patients, and found that effective CPAP treatment compared with sham (or subtherapuetic) CPAP in patients with OSA significantly reduced pulmonary systolic pressure (from 28.9 ± 8.6 to 24.0 ± 5.8, $P < .001$). Those who were mostly likely to respond to therapy were patients with PH at baseline or with left ventricular dysfunction. There are some studies, however, that have shown no significant decrease in pulmonary arterial pressure after either tracheostomy [39,40] or CPAP [41,42]. Based on these data, the effect of treatment of OSA on pulmonary hemodynamics is likely to be beneficial, but larger and more definitive studies are needed.

There are even less data to evaluate the effect of treatment of other sleep-disordered breathing on pulmonary hemodynamics. Sleep-related hypoventilation and hypoxemic syndromes can be treated with supplemental oxygen, but the effect on pulmonary arterial pressure is unknown. In patients with chronic obstructive pulmonary disease, nocturnal oxygen therapy has been shown to result in a small decrease in pulmonary artery pressures but did not alter mortality [43]. A case report found the treatment of primary PH with a double-lung transplant resolved an associated Cheyne-Stokes breathing (CSB) pattern [44]. Clearly further studies are required in this area.

PH syndromes associated with sleep-disordered breathing

While SRBDs are commonly considered a mediator in the development of PH, there are not as much data examining the association of sleep-disordered breathing (SDB) occurring as a result of the PH. It has been shown that some types of PH result in particular types of SDB.

Congestive heart failure and SDB

The prognosis of patients with left heart failure with associated PH is worse than that of patients without PH [45]. Left heart failure, resulting in pulmonary venous hypertension, can result in delayed circulation time and a CSB pattern, a form of central sleep apnea. The prevalence of CSB in patients with a left ventricular ejection fraction less than 40% ranges from 25% to 40%. The delayed circulation time and an increased hypercapnic ventilatory response with hyperventilation-induced hypocapnia contribute to the development of periodic breathing [46,47]. This type of breathing pattern has been shown to portend a poorer prognosis, but a recent study did not show that treating the CSB with CPAP improved mortality [48].

PPH and SDB

In one series of 20 patients with primary PH, 30% of patients were found to have periodic breathing [49]. In another series of only 13 patients, 77% had significant nocturnal desaturations [10]. In patients with primary PH, the increased pulmonary artery pressure and pulmonary vascular resistance often result in reduced cardiac output [50]. Together with ventilation-perfusion mismatching, the decreased cardiac output leads to hypoxemia, which may exacerbate periodic breathing patterns.

Summary

SRBDs and PH are inextricably linked, although the mechanisms of association are complex. Physiologic changes associated with SRBDs, including hypoxia, hypercoagulability, and systemic inflammation, may result in alterations in pulmonary hemodynamics. While SDB in and of itself may not result in severe PH, it likely results in elevated pulmonary arterial pressures. Treatment of SDB appears to improve pulmonary arterial pressures. Data are needed to determine if the treatment of SDB will improve clinical outcomes of patients with PH.

References

[1] Barst R, McGoon M, Torbicki A, et al. Diagnosis and differential assessment of pulmonary arterial hypertension. J Am Coll Cardiol 2004; 43(12 Suppl S): 40S–47S.

[2] Hawrylkiewicz I, Sliwinski P, Gorecka D, et al. Pulmonary haemodynamics in patients with OSAS or an overlap syndrome. Monaldi Arch Chest Dis 2004;61(3):148–52.

[3] Niijima M, Kimura H, Edo H, et al. Manifestation of pulmonary hypertension during REM sleep in obstructive sleep apnea syndrome. Am J Respir Crit Care Med 1999;159(6):1766–72.

[4] Alchanatis M, Tourkohoriti G, Kakouros S, et al. Daytime pulmonary hypertension in patients with obstructive sleep apnea: the effect of continuous positive airway pressure on pulmonary hemodynamics. Respiration 2001;68(6):566–72.

[5] Podszus T, Bauer W, Mayer J, et al. Sleep apnea and pulmonary hypertension. Klin Wochenschr 1986;64(3):131–4.

[6] Weitzenblum E, Krieger J, Apprill M, et al. Daytime pulmonary hypertension in patients with obstructive sleep apnea syndrome. Am Rev Respir Dis 1988;138(2):345–9.

[7] Chaouat A, Weitzenblum E, Krieger J, et al. Pulmonary hemodynamics in the obstructive sleep apnea syndrome. Results in 220 consecutive patients. Chest 1996;109(2):380–6.

[8] Bady E, Achkar A, Pascal S, et al. Pulmonary arterial hypertension in patients with sleep apnoea syndrome. Thorax 2000;55(11):934–9.

[9] Atwood CW Jr, McCrory D, Garcia JG, et al. Pulmonary artery hypertension and sleep-disordered breathing: ACCP evidence-based clinical practice guidelines. Chest 2004;126(1 Suppl): 72S–7S.

[10] Rafanan AL, Golish JA, Dinner DS, et al. Nocturnal hypoxemia is common in primary pulmonary hypertension. Chest 2001;120(3):894–9.

[11] Zielinski J. Effects of intermittent hypoxia on pulmonary haemodynamics: animal models versus studies in humans. Eur Respir J 2005;25(1): 173–80.

[12] Laks L, Lehrhaft B, Grunstein RR, et al. Pulmonary hypertension in obstructive sleep apnoea. Eur Respir J 1995;8(4):537–41.

[13] Weir EK, Reeve HL, Johnson G, et al. A role for potassium channels in smooth muscle cells and platelets in the etiology of primary pulmonary hypertension. Chest 1998;114(3 Suppl): 200S–4S.

[14] Post JM, Hume JR, Archer SL, et al. Direct role for potassium channel inhibition in hypoxic pulmonary vasoconstriction. Am J Physiol 1992; 262(4 Pt 1):C882–90.

[15] Dinh-Xuan AT, Higenbottam TW, Clelland CA, et al. Impairment of endothelium-dependent pulmonary-artery relaxation in chronic obstructive lung disease. N Engl J Med 1991;324(22): 1539–47.

[16] Hasleton PS, Heath D, Brewer DB. Hypertensive pulmonary vascular disease in states of chronic hypoxia. J Pathol Bacteriol 1968;95(2):431–40.

[17] Magee F, Wright JL, Wiggs BR, et al. Pulmonary vascular structure and function in chronic obstructive pulmonary disease. Thorax 1988;43(3): 183–9.

[18] Wilkinson M, Langhorne CA, Heath D, et al. A pathophysiological study of 10 cases of hypoxic cor pulmonale. Q J Med 1988;66(249): 65–85.

[19] Calverley PM, Howatson R, Flenley DC, et al. Clinicopathological correlations in cor pulmonale. Thorax 1992;47(7):494–8.

[20] Strohl KP, Altose MD. Oxygen saturation during breath-holding and during apneas in sleep. Chest 1984;85(2):181–6.

[21] Schulz R, Mahmoudi S, Hattar K, et al. Enhanced release of superoxide from polymorphonuclear neutrophils in obstructive sleep apnea. Impact of continuous positive airway pressure therapy. Am J Respir Crit Care Med 2000;162(2 Pt 1): 566–70.

[22] Phillips BG, Narkiewicz K, Pesek CA, et al. Effects of obstructive sleep apnea on endothelin-1 and blood pressure. J Hypertens 1999;17(1):61–6.

[23] Chin K, Nakamura T, Shimizu K, et al. Effects of nasal continuous positive airway pressure on soluble cell adhesion molecules in patients with obstructive sleep apnea syndrome. Am J Med 2000;109(7):562–7.

[24] Ip MS, Lam B, Chan LY, et al. Circulating nitric oxide is suppressed in obstructive sleep apnea and is reversed by nasal continuous positive airway pressure. Am J Respir Crit Care Med 2000; 162(6):2166–71.

[25] McGuire M, Bradford A. Chronic intermittent hypercapnic hypoxia increases pulmonary arterial pressure and haematocrit in rats. Eur Respir J 2001;18(2):279–85.

[26] von Kanel R, Le DT, Nelesen RA, et al. The hypercoagulable state in sleep apnea is related to comorbid hypertension. J Hypertens 2001;19(8): 1445–51.

[27] Bokinsky G, Miller M, Ault K, et al. Spontaneous platelet activation and aggregation during obstructive sleep apnea and its response to therapy with nasal continuous positive airway pressure. A preliminary investigation. Chest 1995; 108(3):625–30.

[28] Nobili L, Schiavi G, Bozano E, et al. Morning increase of whole blood viscosity in obstructive sleep apnea syndrome. Clin Hemorheol Microcirc 2000;22(1):21–7.

[29] Hoffstein V, Herridge M, Mateika S, et al. Hematocrit levels in sleep apnea. Chest 1994;106(3): 787–91.

[30] Chin K, Ohi M, Kita H, et al. Effects of NCPAP therapy on fibrinogen levels in obstructive sleep apnea syndrome. Am J Respir Crit Care Med 1996;153(6 Pt 1):1972–6.

[31] Eisensehr I, Ehrenberg BL, Noachtar S, et al. Platelet activation, epinephrine, and blood pressure in obstructive sleep apnea syndrome. Neurology 1998;51(1):188–95.

[32] Hartmann G, Tschop M, Fischer R, et al. High altitude increases circulating interleukin-6, interleukin-1 receptor antagonist and C-reactive protein. Cytokine 2000;12(3):246–52.

[33] Vgontzas AN, Papanicolaou DA, Bixler EO, et al. Elevation of plasma cytokines in disorders of excessive daytime sleepiness: role of sleep disturbance and obesity. J Clin Endocrinol Metab 1997;82(5):1313–6.

[34] Vgontzas AN, Papanicolaou DA, Bixler EO, et al. Circadian interleukin-6 secretion and quantity

and depth of sleep. J Clin Endocrinol Metab 1999;84(8):2603–7.

[35] Shamsuzzaman AS, Winnicki M, Lanfranchi P, et al. Elevated C-reactive protein in patients with obstructive sleep apnea. Circulation 2002; 105(21):2462–4.

[36] Kasasbeh E, Chi DS, Krishnaswamy G. Inflammatory aspects of sleep apnea and their cardiovascular consequences. South Med J 2006;99(1): 58–67.

[37] Fletcher EC, Miller J, Schaaf JW, et al. Urinary catecholamines before and after tracheostomy in patients with obstructive sleep apnea and hypertension. Sleep 1987;10(1):35–44.

[38] Arias MA, Garcia-Rio F, Alonso-Fernandez A, et al. Pulmonary hypertension in obstructive sleep apnoea: effects of continuous positive airway pressure: a randomized, controlled crossover study. Eur Heart J 2006;27(9):1106–13.

[39] Coccagna G, Mantovani M, Brignani F, et al. Tracheostomy in hypersomnia with periodic breathing. Bull Physiopathol Respir (Nancy) 1972;8(5): 1217–27.

[40] Fletcher EC, Schaaf JW, Miller J, et al. Long-term cardiopulmonary sequelae in patients with sleep apnea and chronic lung disease. Am Rev Respir Dis 1987;135(3):525–33.

[41] Sforza E, Krieger J, Weitzenblum E, et al. Long-term effects of treatment with nasal continuous positive airway pressure on daytime lung function and pulmonary hemodynamics in patients with obstructive sleep apnea. Am Rev Respir Dis 1990;141(4 Pt 1):866–70.

[42] Chaouat A, Weitzenblum E, Kessler R, et al. Five-year effects of nasal continuous positive airway pressure in obstructive sleep apnoea syndrome. Eur Respir J 1997;10(11):2578–82.

[43] Chaouat A, Weitzenblum E, Kessler R, et al. A randomized trial of nocturnal oxygen therapy in chronic obstructive pulmonary disease patients. Eur Respir J 1999;14:1002–8.

[44] Schulz R, Fegbeutel C, Olschewski H, et al. Reversal of nocturnal periodic breathing in primary pulmonary hypertension after lung transplantation. Chest 2004;125(1):344–7.

[45] Abramson SV, Burke JF, Kelly JJ Jr, et al. Pulmonary hypertension predicts mortality and morbidity in patients with dilated cardiomyopathy. Ann Intern Med 1992;116(11):888–95.

[46] Fanfulla F, Mortara A, Maestri R, et al. The development of hyperventilation in patients with chronic heart failure and Cheyne-Strokes respiration: a possible role of chronic hypoxia. Chest 1998;114(4):1083–90.

[47] Mortara A, Bernardi L, Pinna GD, et al. Alterations of breathing in chronic heart failure: clinical relevance of arterial oxygen saturation instability. Clin Sci (Lond) 1996;91(Suppl): 72–4.

[48] Bradley T, Logan A, Kimoff J, et al. CPAP for central sleep apnea and heart failure. N Engl J Med 2005;353(19):2025–33.

[49] Schulz R, Baseler G, Ghofrani HA, et al. Nocturnal periodic breathing in primary pulmonary hypertension. Eur Respir J 2002;19(4): 658–63.

[50] Javaheri S, Parker TJ, Wexler L, et al. Occult sleep-disordered breathing in stable congestive heart failure. Ann Intern Med 1995;122(7): 487–92.

Special Article

SLEEP
MEDICINE
CLINICS

Sleep Med Clin 2 (2007) 107–117

Sleep-Related Breathing Disorder and Heart Disease—Central Sleep Apnea

Timothy A. Connolly, MD[a], Amir Sharafkhaneh, MD[b,c],*

Overview

Cardiovascular disease is the principal cause of morbidity and mortality in industrialized nations. Congestive heart failure (CHF), in particular, is the leading reason for hospitalization in people over 65 years of age in the United States. Not surprisingly, CHF also is the most common diagnosis-related group encountered in clinical practice; more Centers for Medicare and Medicaid Services (CMS) dollars are spent on CHF than on any other condition, accounting for more than 5% of the national health care budget [1]. In recent years, many advances have occurred in the treatment of CHF with increasing use of specific medications such as beta-adrenergic receptor antagonists, angiotensin-converting enzyme inhibitors, and spironolactone, with resultant decreases in morbidity and mortality [2–4]. Despite enhanced pharmacologic treatment, however, mortality associated with systolic CHF still remains significantly elevated at 50% at 5 years [5].

Sleep-related breathing disorder (SRBD) is a general term encompassing both obstructive sleep apnea (OSA) and central sleep apnea (CSA). Sleep-disordered breathing is being recognized increasingly as a major public health concern. OSA results from complete or partial upper airway obstruction, whereas CSA generally arises from a reduction in overall respiratory drive. The Wisconsin-based cohort study of state employees younger than 65 years of age found the prevalence of sleep-disordered breathing, defined as an apnea-hypopnea index

[a] Baylor College of Medicine, Pulmonary/Critical Care Section, 2002 Holcombe Blvd., Houston, TX 77030, USA
[b] Veterans Affairs Medical Center, 6624 Fannin, Suite 1730, Houston, TX 77030, USA
[c] Baylor College of Medicine, 2002 Holcombe Blvd., Houston, TX 77030, USA
* Corresponding author. MED VAMC Sleep Center (111i), 2002 Holcombe Blvd., Bldg. 100, Rm 6C344, Houston, TX 77030.
E-mail address: amirs@bcm.tmc.edu (A. Sharafkhaneh).

doi:10.1016/j.jsmc.2007.01.001

(AHI) greater than five events per hour, to be 9% in women and 24% in men [6]. In recent years, many studies have demonstrated significant associations between sleep-disordered breathing and multiple cardiovascular disease processes including systemic hypertension, pulmonary hypertension, coronary artery disease, cerebrovascular accidents, and arrhythmias [7–11]. In particular, SRBD, including both OSA and CSA, has been shown to coexist commonly with systolic CHF.

A significant limitation to the current practice guidelines for the chronic care of CHF is the focus on the patient only during waking hours. The supposition that the cardiopulmonary disease processes are dormant during sleep and are not impacted significantly by potential comorbid conditions such as sleep-disordered breathing underestimates the complexity of CHF [12]. Unrecognized disruptions to the already heterogeneous physiology of sleep such as oxygen desaturations and arousals leading to increased sympathetic nervous system activity point to a negative impact on overall cardiovascular disease pathogenesis as well as to a potential novel intervention for improving patient care. Unfortunately, in the clinical management of CHF, SRBD remains a much under diagnosed comorbid entity.

This article reviews cardiovascular physiology and ventilatory control during sleep, the epidemiology of SRBD in CHF, the pathophysiology of CSA as it relates to CHF, and the clinical features and implications of SRBD in systolic CHF. It then focuses on treatment options for CHF-related CSA including continuous positive airway pressure (CPAP) and newer modalities such as adaptive pressure support servo-ventilation (ASV).

Definitions

Before proceeding with a more detailed discussion of sleep-disordered breathing and its clinical association with systolic CHF, it is important to define some operational polysomnographic (PSG) terms. Apnea, in adults, is the absence of airflow detected at the nose or mouth for longer than 10 seconds [13]. The type of apnea is further classified by inspiratory effort. An obstructive apnea is the absence of tidal volume with continued respiratory effort as measured by thoracoabdominal bands [14]. By contrast, a central apnea is the absence of tidal volume with a complete absence of respiratory effort. Obstructive hypopnea has a variety of definitions, but the one currently adopted by CMS and by most practicing sleep laboratories is a reduction in airflow of 30% from baseline for longer than 10 seconds with an associated oxygen desaturation more

than or equal to 4%. Of note, arousals, which may play a disruptive role in the pathogenesis of systolic CHF, are not considered in the definition of CMS hypopnea [14]. The AHI is the total number of apneas and hypopneas divided by total sleep time and is expressed as the number of events per hour. AHI serves as the most commonly used objective clinical measure of sleep apnea severity. Although various criteria have been used in research protocols, it is generally accepted that CSA syndrome is an AHI greater than five events per hour with more than 50% of the respiratory events classified as central rather than obstructive [11]. Cheyne-Stokes respiration (CSR) is a subtype of CSA constituted by periodic breathing in which central apneas (and hypopneas) alternate with periods of hyperventilation in a crescendo/decrescendo ventilatory pattern. Even though it is classically taught that CSA-CSR is found most commonly in association with systolic CHF, it is important to remember that the majority of patients who have central apneas also have some obstructive physiology, and vice versa.

Cardiovascular physiology during sleep

The principal impact of various stages of sleep on the cardiovascular system stems from the respective level of autonomic nervous system activity. In normal subjects, non–rapid eye movement (NREM) sleep is a state of general cardiovascular and hemodynamic relaxation under increasing parasympathetic influence. Heart rate, blood pressure, systemic vascular resistance, cardiac output, and metabolic activity are reduced with higher vagal activity [15]. In rapid eye movement (REM) sleep, even though transient phasic bursts of sympathetic activity occur, the average heart rate and blood pressure remain below waking levels [16].

Increased parasympathetic activity during NREM sleep is thought to suppress the development of cardiac rhythm disturbances, whereas sympathetic surges during REM are believed to facilitate ventricular arrhythmias. Similarly, phasic REM sympathetic discharges also may predispose patients who have underlying atherosclerotic coronary artery stenosis to nocturnal angina because rapid heart rates allow decreased diastolic coronary perfusion time [17].

Normal physiologic responses to arousal from sleep include activation of the sympathetic nervous system with associated increases in heart rate and blood pressure and decreased overall parasympathetic activity. Patients who have SRBD often have multiple recurrent episodes of inadequate breathing leading to respiratory-related arousals, often with concomitant oxygen desaturation. These multiple stressors can apply additional strain on an already vulnerable cardiovascular system in patients who have depressed left ventricular ejection fractions (LVEF).

Ventilatory control during sleep

Ventilation is considered to be the main function of breathing and therefore is the primary target of control by the central nervous system. Regulation of ventilation is a complex process involving interaction of the involuntary metabolic processes at the brainstem level along with the voluntary control mechanisms in the cortex influenced by the level of arousal. The metabolic control systems involve feedback from stretch and irritant receptors in the lung as well as both central and peripheral chemoreceptors. Central chemoreceptors use CO_2 and cerebrospinal fluid pH in the medullary brainstem centers, whereas peripheral chemoreceptors recognize both Pa_{O_2} and to a lesser extent Pa_{CO_2} levels through the carotid and aortic bodies.

Under normal circumstances, whenever arterial Pa_{CO_2} rises, ventilation is stimulated to bring Pa_{CO_2} back to the previous steady state level. This process is termed the "hypercapnic ventilatory response." During wakefulness, a voluntary "wake drive" allows the maintenance of tidal volume even if the Pa_{CO_2} falls below the eucapnic wake level to an apnea threshold that otherwise might reduce the respiratory drive and lead to the development of CSA [18]. During NREM sleep, because this voluntary control is lost, the metabolic control systems become even more critical. Sleep onset itself leads to decreased sensitivity of the chemoreceptors and a blunting of the hypercapnic ventilatory response. When coupled with decreased upper airway caliber and increased airflow resistance, this phenomenon generally causes a normal rise in Pa_{CO_2} to a eucapnic sleep level that is 4 to 6 mm Hg above the eucapnic wake level. During REM sleep, ventilation normally has irregular periods, especially during phasic eye bursts. The chemosensitivity of the ventilatory system in REM is recognized to be even lower than in NREM sleep, which results in further CO_2 elevation. While sleeping, men have a more diminished responsiveness to CO_2 than women and therefore are more susceptible to the development of CSA [19].

Classification of central sleep apnea

CSA can be divided into two general categories based on an understanding of this background physiology. Hypercapnic CSA results from a decreased sensitivity of the chemoreceptors superimposed on a loss of the voluntary "wake drive"

which together result in an overall reduction in respiratory drive [20]. This hypoventilation is exaggerated by progressively decreased chemosensitivity as the individual transitions from NREM to REM sleep. Clinically this phenomenon manifests as alveolar hypoventilation syndromes, examples of which include the obesity-hypoventilation syndrome, neuromuscular failure, chronic narcotic use, and idiopathic central hypoventilation (also known as "Ondine's curse"). These individuals normally are recognized as chronic CO_2 retainers and in many cases require some form of mechanical ventilatory support.

Nonhypercapnic CSA, by contrast, results from increased sensitivity of the chemoreceptors leading to robust ventilatory responses to even trivial changes in Pa_{CO_2}. During NREM sleep, hyperventilation can drive Pa_{CO_2} below the apnea threshold, which generally is 2 to 6 mm Hg below the eucapnic sleep level, causing cessation of respiratory effort and airflow [18]. Subsequent elevation of Pa_{CO_2}, caused by the apnea, again triggers ventilation, and the cycle repeats. During REM sleep, as Pa_{CO_2} normally rises even higher than NREM levels, the separation between the eucapnic sleep level and the apnea threshold increases, making it harder to hyperventilate down below the apnea threshold. This increase in Pa_{CO_2} serves to stabilize the ventilatory control systems and explains why CSA events are rarely seen during REM sleep. Examples of conditions associated with nonhypercapnic CSA include CSR in systolic CHF, periodic breathing at high altitude, sleep transition states, and the initiation of CPAP therapy. These individuals (with nonhypercapnic CSA) have normal or even low baseline daytime Pa_{CO_2} on arterial blood gas analysis.

Epidemiology of sleep-related breathing disorder in congestive heart failure

As mentioned earlier, SRBD is common in patients who have systolic CHF. In fact, the overall likelihood of sleep-disordered breathing in patients who have an LVEF of less than 45% is estimated to be at least 45% [21]. In patients who have systolic CHF, OSA has a prevalence of 11% to 37%, and CSA is even more common, with a prevalence of 33% to 40% [11,22]. In the Sleep Heart Health Study, the presence of OSA (defined by an AHI > 11 events per hour) carried a 2.38 greater relative risk of the patient's having associated CHF regardless of additional known predisposing features [8]. Risk factors for OSA in this CHF group also differed by gender: in men, obesity with a body mass index greater than 35 was the main predictor, whereas in women an age greater than 60 years was the key feature [11].

Fewer studies are available that examine the prevalence of CSA specifically in patients who have systolic CHF. The four major risk factors for the presence of CSA, identified by Sin and colleagues [11] in a retrospective analysis of PSG studies in 450 men and women who had CHF, included male gender, age greater than 60 years, transcutaneous Pco_2 less than 30 mm Hg, and atrial fibrillation. In the largest prospective study to date on this topic, Javaheri and colleagues [22] performed PSG on 81 ambulatory men who had stable systolic CHF. They found that the presence of CSA was inversely related to the LVEF but was not predicted by the New York Heart Association (NYHA) classification score.

Central sleep apnea in congestive heart failure

Pathophysiology

CSA probably is a consequence of CHF and serves as another clinical marker for suboptimal cardiovascular function. Its presence should alert the physician to the need for intensifying treatment. Patients who have CHF and who are not fully compensated have chronic hyperventilation driven by stimulation of the lung's vagal irritant receptors caused by elevated pulmonary venous congestion as well as by the increased sensitivity of central and peripheral chemoreceptors [12]. Lying supine during sleep mobilizes additional fluid into the central circulation, worsening vascular congestion and further decreasing lung compliance. Additionally, transient apnea-induced hypoxia also contributes to a given patient's tendency for hyperventilation.

If volume overload is indeed the cause of chronic hyperventilation in CHF, it follows that elevated pulmonary capillary wedge pressures (PCWP) correlates with the presence of CSA. Solin and colleagues [23] evaluated 75 stable patients who had CHF with right heart catheterization to investigate this relationship further. Most of the participants were in NYHA class III with a mean LVEF of 20%. The patients then were categorized into three groups based on overnight PSG findings: those who had no apnea (n = 22), those who had OSA (n = 20), and those who had CSA (n = 33). The CSA group had a significantly higher PCWP (22.8 ± 1.2) than the no-apnea (11.5 ± 1.3) and the OSA (12.3 ± 1.2) groups ($P<.001$), and treatment directed at reducing the PCWP resulted in significantly fewer total CSA events.

Recall that nonhypercapnic CSA occurs when hyperventilation leads to a reduction in the $Paco_2$ from the eucapnic sleep level to below the apnea threshold. Apnea then persists until the $Paco_2$ rises and again triggers ventilation in a repetitive cycle. Unlike with obstructive events, arousals are not required for initiation of airflow at the termination of central apneas, but nonetheless arousals often do occur at the peak of inspiratory effort. Even though the inspiratory effort is not as severe as that measured when patients are forced to breath against an obstructed upper airway, the increased inspiratory effort between apneas during CSA leads to more negative intrathoracic pressure swings and subsequent elevation of left ventricular (LV) afterload, which clearly is detrimental to CHF control [24].

The pathophysiology for nonhypercapnic CSA was elucidated further in a 1999 article by Lorenzi-Filho and associates [25]. Ten patients who had CSA and LVEF ranging from 9% to 31% were studied after inhaling gas mixtures composed of either room air or 4% CO_2. The individuals who inhaled the CO_2-enriched gas had a significant reduction in CSA events as a percentage of total sleep time when compared with those who breathed the room air mixture, 19% versus 40% ($P<.003$). The findings indicate that inhalation of a CO_2-enhanced gas with resultant elevation in $Paco_2$ has the ability to abolish CSA, although it is not necessarily a clinically practical treatment option. This concept lends further validity to the observation that fewer nonhypercapnic CSA events occur during REM sleep, which is effectively a "CO_2-enriched state," than in NREM sleep .

Clinical Presentation

It is not clear whether specific clinical features exist for CSA. Although sleep fragmentation caused by recurrent arousals often disrupts the sleep architecture on formal PSG testing, most patients who have CHF with CSA do not complain of habitual snoring or excessive daytime sleepiness [22]. Orthopnea and paroxysmal nocturnal dyspnea actually may be clinical representations of arousals that occur during the peak hyperpneic respiratory phase of a central apnea rather than simply a manifestation of unstable pulmonary venous congestion. As mentioned earlier, men are more predisposed to CSA than women. It is intriguing to speculate whether this difference may explain, in part, gender differences seen in CHF mortality [26].

Obviously many patients who have CSA have concomitant OSA, making the overlap of clinical features quite possible. In these patients there is often a gradual transition from obstructive events early in the sleep period to predominantly central events later on. It is believed that this shift results from both a prolongation in circulation time and a reduction in $Paco_2$ toward the apnea threshold [27].

It has been shown previously that patients who have CHF and SRBD have significantly lower LVEFs than similar matched cohorts who do not have concomitant SRBD, 22% versus 27% (*P*<.01). Even though there was no statistical difference in body mass index, both AHI and arousals were significantly elevated in patients who had SRBD, and the arterial oxygen saturation nadir was significantly lower, 76% versus 89% (*P*<.05), than in patients who did not have SRBD [22].

Garrigue and his cardiology colleagues [28] observed an interesting clinical experience in some of their patients who had CHF with comorbid SRBD. Individuals who had received a pacemaker to treat tachyarrhythmias or symptomatic bradycardia reported a reduction in breathing disorders after implantation of the device. Fifteen patients who had SRBD (73% of whom had concomitant systolic CHF, but only one of whom had classic CSA-CSR) were evaluated for improvements in sleep parameters after pacemaker placement. After a first night for baseline PSG, two additional evenings were spent in the sleep laboratory, in random order, with the pacemaker programmed either to spontaneous mode (ventricular rate of 40 beats/minute), or atrial overdrive pacing (15 beats/minute faster than the patient's mean nocturnal sinus rate). With atrial overdrive pacing reduction of more than 50% in the AHI was achieved in 87% of the patients, regardless of whether they had predominantly OSA or CSA. Subsequent confirmatory studies have had mixed results [29–32], including recent work by the authors' own group in 15 elderly male veterans who had a mean LVEF of 38% and obstructive AHI of 35 events per hour. Significant improvement was observed in the apnea index with atrial overdrive pacing, but no differences in AHI, minimum O_2, or average O_2 saturations were seen [33]. The mechanisms behind any amelioration of sleep-disordered breathing by this overdrive pacing are not fully understood, but the results emphasize the important interplay between the nocturnal respiratory system and cardiovascular function.

Clinical Implications

CSA-CSR in systolic CHF is associated with increased mortality [34]. As explained already, CSA generally indicates suboptimal medical control of CHF, so the correlation with worse clinical outcomes should come as no surprise. Of increasing clinical interest, however, is the proposal that CSA itself may contribute directly to a progressive deterioration of cardiac status. Proposed mechanisms for the negative cardiac pathogenesis associated with CSA generally focus on electroencephalographic arousals with or without hypoxemia leading to significantly increased sympathetic nervous system activity.

To determine the prognostic value of CSA in CHF, Lanfranchi and associates [35] followed 54 patients who had CHF for a mean period of 28 months. Thirty-nine survivors were compared with 15 non-survivors in categories such as NYHA class, peak oxygen consumption (Vo_2) on cardiopulmonary exercise testing, LVEF, left atrial area size, central AHI, and percentage of total sleep time spent with arterial oxygen saturation below 90%. The highest risk for death was determined to be a central AHI greater than 30 events per hour and left atrial size greater than 25 cm^2.

Increased sympathetic nervous system activity (SNSA) in patients who have CHF is a marker of ongoing cardiovascular stress and is associated clearly with detrimental outcomes [36]. SRBD itself also leads to elevated SNSA activity, but the mechanisms are slightly different in OSA than in CSA. Obstruction of the upper airway often causes oxygen desaturation and requires an arousal to open the airway before airflow will resume. Both these features result in transient elevation of SNSA occurring at the termination of an obstructive event. Alternatively, CSA may or may not involve hypoxia, and arousals, when present, usually manifest at the peak of ventilation during the postapnea hyperpneic phase. In contrast to OSA, SNSA elevation in CSA persists during the waking hours as well, consistent with a more disturbed overall state of cardiac function [37]. As a result of tonic sympathetic nervous stimulation, patients may develop decreased heart rate variability and malignant ventricular arrhythmias.

Lanfranchi and colleagues [38] examined 47 patients who did not have known CHF who coincidentally were found to have an LVEF of less than 40% by screening echocardiography on presentation to a cardiology clinic. CSA was found to be highly prevalent (55%) in these asymptomatic individuals who had LV dysfunction. It is expected that this prevalence would be higher than values previously reported because none of these patients had yet received appropriate medical therapy for CHF. In addition, patients who had CSA also were noted to have markedly decreased heart rate variability (*P*<.05) as well as an increased incidence of daytime nonsustained ventricular tachycardia. Both of these developments serve as markers for increased cardiovascular morbidity and mortality in the context of underlying systolic CHF [39].

Indications for sleep studies in congestive heart failure

Recently published practice parameters from the American Academy of Sleep Medicine [40] offer guidance in regard to the indications for ordering

PSG in patients who have CHF. Based on a number of good-quality studies, the committee was able to make the following standard recommendation, which currently is regarded as the generally accepted patient-care strategy: "Patients with systolic (or diastolic) heart failure should undergo polysomnography if they have symptoms suggestive of sleep-related breathing disorders (disturbed sleep, nocturnal dyspnea, snoring) or if they remain symptomatic despite optimal medical management of congestive heart failure." Other clinical clues, not mentioned in the guidelines, that also may prompt the sleep specialist to order a PSG to investigate further the presence of CSA in CHF include excess premature ventricular beats (> 30/hour) and couplets, nonsustained ventricular tachycardia, and atrial fibrillation [41].

Treatment

To Treat or not to Treat?

The ultimate goals for addressing CSA in systolic CHF are improvement of cardiovascular function, enhanced quality of life, and possibly even reduced morbidity and mortality. Unfortunately, at present, there is no consensus as to whether CSA should be treated directly, let alone what the ideal approach might involve [12]. The foundation for any successful treatment strategy targeting nonhypercapnic CSA is, first and foremost, maximization of medical therapy for CHF. As has been shown already, CSA may not act simply as a passive marker for CHF. Because of fragmented sleep, arousals, hypoxia, and unwanted excessive SNSA, CSA-CSR that persists despite optimal pharmacologic treatment probably should be approached aggressively. Multiple adjunctive therapeutic options, with varying levels of supporting evidence, are available (eg, supplemental nocturnal oxygen, medications, and various forms of noninvasive positive airway pressure).

Most of the studies of CSA reviewed thus far were conducted before the current standard medical therapy for CHF became widespread. Accordingly, mortality projections recently have underestimated how much benefit has been achieved during the last 10 years with regular incorporation of beta-blockers, angiotensin-converting enzyme inhibitors, and spironolactone into the pharmaceutical arsenal. However, just because a given treatment makes sense for the treatment of CHF, it does not mean that it also will have a positive impact on CSA. For example, diuresis in CHF obviously helps decrease pulmonary congestion, thereby improving dyspnea scores and exercise tolerance, but overdiuresis may, in fact, result in iatrogenic metabolic alkalosis that can worsen CSA. Accordingly, the limited or preliminary data for many of the treatment options available to clinicians today make full endorsement difficult.

Treatment Options

Supplemental oxygen

Supplemental O_2 seems to be a logical choice for addressing apnea-related hypoxia in patients who have CHF and comorbid CSA, but controversy currently exists as to its utility and safety. A number of experts favor nocturnal O_2 as a treatment for CSA. O_2 is known to raise $Paco_2$, by the Haldane effect, thereby increasing the difference between the eucapnic sleep level and the apnea threshold. Just as is seen with the transition from NREM to REM sleep, this separation results in fewer nonhypercapnic CSA events. O_2 also has been noted to decrease arousals and shift sleep to deeper stages, resulting in improved overall sleep architecture and reduced SNSA [42–44]. Opponents of O_2 supplementation explain that no long-term trials have demonstrated that the use of nocturnal O_2 improves the natural clinical history of CHF. Some investigators even raise theoretical concerns about cardiodepressant and proinflammatory vascular effects by oxidant free radicals [45]. Despite its ease of administration, clinicians still await long-term outcome data to determine the ultimate role of nocturnal supplemental nasal O_2 as therapy for CSA in CHF [46].

Acetazolamide

Acetazolamide is a mild diuretic that has long been employed as a respiratory stimulant in the treatment of nonhypercapnic CSA caused by periodic breathing at high altitude. By creating a metabolic acidosis and an increased stimulus to breathe, acetazolamide causes the $Paco_2$ level to fall, but the apneic threshold falls even further [47]. Because the difference between the new eucapnic sleep level and apnea threshold actually increases, fewer CSA events are observed. A recent double-blind, crossover protocol examined 12 male patients who had stable systolic CHF (mean LVEF, 19%) and a central AHI greater than 15. Patients received acetazolamide, 3.5 mg/kg, 1 hour before bedtime for 6 nights versus placebo with a 2-week washout period. The target goal was a reduction in CO_2 by 5 mmol/L. Significant improvements were noted in patients during the period of acetazolamide administration with a reduced CSA index of 23 events per hour versus 49 events per hour ($P = .004$) and a reduced percentage of total sleep time spent with Spo_2 below 90%, 6% versus 19% ($P = .01$) [48]. Larger trials are needed before this medication can be recommended as a standard chronic treatment for CSA in CHF.

Theophylline

Another known central respiratory stimulant, theophylline, similarly has been investigated for use in this patient population. Fifteen men who had LVEFs of less than 45% were followed using a double-blind, crossover format comparing twice daily theophylline versus placebo for 5 days [49]. Although theophylline reduced central AHI, the desaturation index, and electroencephalographic arousals, significant concern still exists about the safety profile of this agent in CHF. Potential adverse consequences of the methylxanthine family, such as inotropic stimulation and arrhythmogenesis, preclude the chronic use of this drug in advanced systolic heart failure at present [12].

Positive airway pressure

Positive pressure ventilation has long been recognized in the ICU setting to have beneficial effects on depressed cardiac pump function whether encountered postoperatively after open-heart surgery or during acute exacerbations of CHF [50]. Naughton and colleagues [51] confirmed these hemodynamic benefits in 15 patients who had systolic CHF and nine "normal" patients, while awake, using real-time echocardiography. Nasal CPAP, similar to that used for the routine treatment of OSA, was administered using pressures ranging from 0 to 10 cm H_2O. Positive airway pressure increased intrathoracic pressures with resultant reductions in both venous return and LV transmural pressure. Clinical correlates of these physiologic parameters include both decreased cardiac preload and LV afterload. The acute impact is generally enhanced systolic function.

Overnight measurement of urinary norepinephrine (UNE) levels has been shown previously to serve as a consistent marker of integrated SNSA during sleep [31]. In another study, Naughton and colleagues [52] followed 35 patients who had systolic CHF divided into two groups based on the presence or absence of CSA. Seventeen patients who had no CSA recorded a baseline UNE level of 16 nmol/mmol of creatinine. The 18 patients who had CSA began with a UNE level significantly higher at 30 nmol/mmol ($P<.005$). After treatment with nasal CPAP over a 1-month period, the patients who did not have CSA had a reduction in UNE to -1.3; the CSA group manifested an even more dramatic decline to -12.5 ($P<.025$). Despite clear physiologic improvements from CPAP, questions still remained about clinically relevant long-term outcomes in patients who have CHF and comorbid SRBD.

Early work by the Toronto group showed that in patients who have CHF with comorbid OSA, LV afterload increases as the patients transitioned from wake to stage 2 NREM sleep. CPAP abolished obstructive events and thereby reduced LV afterload and heart rate, unloaded muscles of respiration, and improved oxygenation during NREM sleep [53]. In 2003, Kaneko, and colleagues [54] published a study again highlighting the cardiovascular effects of CPAP therapy in patients who had CHF and comorbid OSA. Twenty-four patients who had advanced systolic dysfunction (mean ejection fraction of 25%) and moderate-to-severe OSA (AHI > 20 events per hour) were assigned randomly to continue maximal medical therapy with or without nasal CPAP for 1 month. In addition to reduced daytime systolic blood pressure, heart rate, and LV end systolic dimensions, sustained improvements were noted also in LVEF. Regular CPAP use for 1 month, in addition to maximal medical CHF therapy resulted in a 9% absolute and a 35% relative increase in LVEF for patients who had systolic CHF with concomitant OSA. Whether these improvements will be sustainable beyond 1 month has yet to be examined, but the role of positive airway pressure as an adjunctive treatment for patients who have systolic CHF and comorbid OSA seems reasonable.

A similar pilot project conducted a few years earlier by Sin and colleagues [55] focused instead on CPAP therapy for patients who had systolic CHF and comorbid CSA. Sixty-six patients were enrolled and assigned randomly to continue "maximal" medical therapy alone or to have nasal CPAP, 10 to 12.5 cm H_2O, administered nightly for 3 months. The patients were followed subsequently for 2 years. The 29 patients who had CSA manifested an 8% improvement in LVEF at 3 months. There also was a dramatic relative risk reduction of 81% in the combined mortality-cardiac transplantation rate at 2 years. Trial enrollment occurred before the widespread use of beta-blockers as treatment for CHF, however, so the maximal medical therapy at that time does not necessarily reflect the current standard in 2007.

The recently completed multicenter Canadian Positive Airway Pressure (CANPAP) trial evaluated 258 patients who had CHF with advanced but stable cardiac disease (mean LVEF, 25%) [56]. These individuals also had clinically significant sleep-disordered breathing with mean AHI of 40 events per hour, 90% of which were central events. Investigators wanted to test the hypothesis that long-term treatment of CSA with CPAP, in patients who have systolic CHF and are simultaneously receiving optimal medical therapy, reduces the combined rates of death and cardiac transplantation. CPAP was given initially to 128 patients starting at a level of 5 cm H_2O and subsequently titrated, in a monitored setting, to a target pressure of 10 cm H_2O or the highest pressure tolerated. The average CPAP pressure used, during the 2-year trial, was 8 to 9 cm H_2O. Although patients were instructed to use the CPAP device at home for more than 6 hours per night, actual usage fell significantly short of that goal, with average times of 4.3 hours per night during the first 3 months and only 3.6 hours per night after 1 year.

The CANPAP trial was terminated prematurely after an interim analysis revealed that the transplant-free survival curve favored the control group. Investigators also recognized that the study was underpowered to achieve statistical significance for the primary endpoint, combined rate of death and cardiac transplantation. An overestimation of the anticipated death-transplantation rate was attributed to the significant improvements in drug therapy for CHF from 1998 to 2004. In particular, 77% of the enrollees in this trial were taking beta-blockers, compared with fewer than 20% in earlier studies [56].

CPAP was shown to yield multiple positive effects such as attenuation of CSA events, improved nocturnal oxygenation, increased LVEF, and lower plasma norepinephrine levels. Even though these physiologic effects were sustained on a long-term basis, there was no difference in the "hard" endpoints, including all-cause mortality, transplant-free survival, and number of hospitalizations, in those who used CPAP and those who relied solely on medical therapy. The authors concluded, "although the CANPAP trial ultimately lacked the power to conclude with certainty that CPAP is ineffective in this patient population; our data do not support its routine use to extend life in patients with CSA and CHF" [56]. Overall, the inconclusive outcome data for CPAP therapy in CSA-CSR and equivalent results achieved with bilevel ventilation [57] have prompted investigators to explore novel modes of ventilatory support.

Adaptive pressure support servo-ventilation

ASV provides a background positive end-expiratory pressure (PEEP) of 4 to 5 cm H_2O with superimposed inspiratory pressure support of 3 to 10 cm H_2O. Ventilation is then servo controlled, based on detection of prolonged CSA events, with a back-up respiratory rate to equal a moving target ventilation of 90% of the subject's long-term average ventilation. Following an apnea, if the patient resumes normal spontaneous respiratory effort and the ventilation continues to exceed the 90% target, support is reduced to a PEEP of 4 cm H_2O. Smaller or slower changes in respiratory effort from steady state result in proportionally smaller, slower changes in the degree of ASV support. The mean airway pressure usually obtained is approximately 7 cm H_2O [58].

In 2001, Teschler and associates [58] compared the acute effects of ASV on sleep quality and breathing with nocturnal supplemental O_2, nasal CPAP, and bilevel ventilation plus back-up rate set at two breaths per minute less than the patient's wake spontaneous respiratory rate. Fourteen subjects who had stable systolic CHF and predominantly CSA-CSR were included in this prospective, randomized, crossover design. For each patient, an in-laboratory baseline PSG was followed by four sequential treatment nights studied in random order with O_2 (2 L/minute by nasal cannulae), nasal CPAP (mean overnight pressure 8.7 ± 0.1 cm H_2O), bilevel ventilation (mean overnight inspiratory positive airway pressure, 12 ± 0.3 cm H_2O; expiratory positive airway pressure, 5.3 ± 0.1 cm H_2O; and overnight mask pressure, 8 cm H_2O), and ASV (mean pressure, 9 cm H_2O during apneas/hypopneas but 7 cm H_2O for the remainder). All four interventions significantly reduced the central apnea index from a baseline of 35.8 events per hour. This index decreased by 50% with both O_2 (19.7 events per hour) and CPAP (18.5 events per hour), 50% more with bilevel ventilation (8.4 events per hour), and an additional 50% with ASV (3.3 events per hour). The overall arousal index at baseline was elevated (66.7 events per hour). All treatment groups demonstrated significant reductions in sleep fragmentation with the most dramatic improvement in the participants receiving bilevel ventilation (18.4 events per hour) and ASV (16.6 events per hour). Each of the four treatments also produced improvements in the 4% desaturation index with supplemental O_2 and ASV superior to the others. Of 14 participants, 13 found ASV more comfortable than the other ventilatory modes, and one regarded ASV and bilevel comfort to be equivalent. In this pilot study one night of therapy with ASV in CSA-CSR provided an 83% further reduction in central apnea index as compared with CPAP at a similar mean pressure, demonstrated enhanced sleep quality, and was preferred subjectively to other ventilatory modes.

Long-term compliance with and efficacy of ASV versus CPAP in the treatment of CSA-CSR was recently evaluated in a 6-month randomized, prospective, parallel comparison trial conducted at a single French center [59]. Twenty-five men who had an ejection fraction of 30% and CSA of 44 events per hour were assigned randomly to receive either nasal CPAP (mean effective pressure, 8 cm H_2O) or ASV (PEEP = 5 cm H_2O; inspiratory pressure support of 3 to 10 cm H_2O; and a back-up rate set at 15 breaths/minute). The mean pressure generally encountered by these ASV default settings is 7 to 9 cm H_2O. The decrease in central AHI was significantly greater with ASV than with CPAP at both 3 and 6 months. Furthermore, only ASV effectively abolished CSA-CSR with a reduction of central

AHI to less than 10 events per hour. Overall compliance was significantly better with ASV than with CPAP, which decreased over time to less than 4 hours per night. Improved adherence to ASV may be attributed to the bilevel effect of pressure adjustments during respiratory cycles, but it also may reflect the overall effectiveness of treatment [60]. ASV also resulted in a statistically significant increase of 7% in LVEF; no such benefit was observed with CPAP. This lack of cardiovascular improvement with CPAP is in contrast to findings of multiple other studies reviewed earlier in this paper and may be explained by the lower overall airway pressure achieved. As intriguing as these preliminary data are, they must be regarded in the context of a small, single-center trial with results somewhat contradictory to earlier more established work.

Summary

Notwithstanding pharmacologic advances in the treatment of systolic CHF, mortality for this condition remains unacceptably high. Appreciation of the coexistence of SRBD and CHF has led investigators to question the potential contribution of abnormal sleep physiology to the pathogenesis of heart failure. In particular, CSA-CSR, once thought merely to serve as a marker for suboptimal CHF control, is now well recognized to impact cardiac function itself negatively through fragmented sleep architecture, arousals, hypoxemia, and tonically elevated SNSA.

At present, there is no uniformly accepted approach to the treatment of CSA-CSR. Multiple adjunctive therapeutic options, such as supplemental nocturnal O_2, nasal CPAP, and ASV, are available to the sleep clinician; each has varying levels of supporting evidence. In coming years, large, well-designed, multicenter clinical trials are needed to support and encourage novel interventions for these complex disease processes. It is hoped that the final result will be enhanced sleep quality and improved cardiovascular control for patients who have SRBD and advanced systolic heart failure.

References

[1] Hunt HA, Baker DW, Chin MH, et al. ACC/AHA guidelines for the evaluation and management of chronic heart failure in the adult: executive summary: a report of the American College of Cardiology/American heart Association task Force on Practice Guidelines. Circulation 2001; 104:2296–3007.

[2] Packer M, Coats AJ, Fowler MB, et al. Carvedilol Prospective Randomized Cumulative Survival Study Group. Effect of carvedilol on survival in severe chronic heart failure. N Engl J Med 2001; 344:1651–8.

[3] The SOLVD Investigators. Effect on survival in patients with reduced left ventricular ejection fractions and congestive heart failure. N Engl J Med 1991;325:293–302.

[4] Pitt B, Zannad F, Remme WJ, et al. The effect of spironolactone on morbidity and mortality in patients with severe heart failure—RALES. N Engl J Med 1999;341(10):709–17.

[5] Levy D, Kenechaiah S, Larson MG, et al. Long-term trends in the incidence of and survival with heart failure. N Engl J Med 2002;347: 1397–402.

[6] Young T, Palta M, Leder R, et al. The occurrence of sleep disordered breathing among middle aged adults. N Engl J Med 1993;328:1230–5.

[7] Nieto FJ, Young TB, Lind BK, et al. Association of sleep-disordered breathing, sleep apnea, and hypertension in a large community based study. Sleep Heart Health Study. JAMA 2000;283: 1829–36.

[8] Shahar E, Whitney CW, Redline S, et al. Sleep-disordered breathing and cardiovascular disease: cross-sectional results of the Sleep Heart Health Study. Am J Respir Crit Care Med 2001;163: 19–25.

[9] Young T, Peppard P, Palta M, et al. Population-based study of sleep-disordered breathing as a risk factor for hypertension. Arch Intern Med 1997;157:1746–52.

[10] Peppard PE, Young T, Palta M, et al. Prospective study of the association between sleep disordered breathing and hypertension. N Engl J Med 2000;342:1378–84.

[11] Sin DD, Fitzgerald F, Parker JD, et al. Risk factors for central and obstructive sleep apnea in 450 men and women with congestive heart failure. Am J Respir Crit Care Med 1999;160(4): 1101–6.

[12] Bradley TD, Floras JS. Sleep apnea and heart failure—2 part series. Circulation 2003;107:1671–8, 1822–6.

[13] Kryger MH. Monitoring respiratory and cardiac function. In: Kryger MH, Roth T, Dement WC, editors. Principles and practice of sleep medicine. Philadelphia: WB Saunders; 2000. p. 1217–30.

[14] Berry RB. Sleep medicine pearls. 2nd edition. Philadelphia: Hanley & Belfus, Inc.; 2003.

[15] Lorenzi-Filho G, Dajani HR, Leung RS, et al. Entrainment of blood pressure and heart rate oscillations by periodic breathing. Am J Respir Crit Care Med 1999;159:1147–54.

[16] Franklin KA, Sandstrom E, Johansson G, et al. Hemodynamics, cerebral circulation, and oxygen saturation in Cheyne-Stokes respiration. J Appl Physiol 1997;83:1184–91.

[17] Kirby DA, Verrier RL. Differential effects of sleep stage on coronary artery hemodynamic function during stenosis. Physiol Behav 1989;45:1017–20.

[18] Malhotra A, Berry RB, White DP. Central sleep apnea. In: Carney PR, Berry RB, Geyer JD, editors. Clinical sleep disorders. Baltimore (MD): Lippincott Williams & Wilkins; 2005. p. 331–46.

[19] Zhou XS, Shahabuddin S, Zahn BK, et al. Effect of gender on the development of hypocapnic apnea/hypopnea during NREM sleep. J Appl Physiol 2000;89:192–9.

[20] Bradley TD. Crossing the threshold—implications for central sleep apnea. Am J Respir Crit Care Med 2002;165:1203–4.

[21] Javaheri S, Parker TJ, Wexler L, et al. Occult sleep-disordered breathing in stable congestive heart failure. Ann Intern Med 1995;122(7):487–92.

[22] Javaheri S, Parker TJ, Liming JD, et al. Sleep apnea in 81 ambulatory male patients with stable heart failure. Types and their prevalences, consequences, and presentations. Circulation 1998;97:2154–9.

[23] Solin P, Bergin P, Richardson M, et al. Influence of pulmonary capillary wedge pressure on central apnea in heart failure. Circulation 1999;99(12):1574–9.

[24] Naughton M, Bernard D, Tam A, et al. Role of hyperventilation in the pathogenesis of central sleep apneas in patients with congestive heart failure. Am Rev Respir Dis 1993;148(2):330–8.

[25] Lorenzi-Filho G, Rankin F, Bies I, et al. Effects of inhaled carbon dioxide and oxygen on Cheyne-Stokes respiration in patients with heart failure. Am J Respir Crit Care Med 1999;159(5 Pt 1):1490–8.

[26] Simon T, Mary-Krause M, Funck-Brentano C, et al. Sex differences in the prognosis of congestive heart failure: results from the Cardiac Insufficiency Bisoprolol Study (CIBIS II). Circulation 2001;103(3):375–80.

[27] Tkacova R, Niroumand M, Lorenzi-Filho G, et al. Overnight shift from obstructive to central apneas in patients with heart failure: role of PaCO2 and circulatory delay. Circulation 2001;103:238–43.

[28] Garrigue S, Bordier P, Jais P, et al. Benefit of atrial pacing in sleep apnea syndrome. N Engl J Med 2002;346(6):404–12.

[29] Luthje L, Unterberg-Buchwald C, Dajani D, et al. Atrial overdrive pacing in patients with sleep apnea with implanted pacemaker. Am J Respir Crit Care Med 2005;172(1):118–22.

[30] Unterberg-Buchwald C, Luthje L, Szych J, et al. Atrial overdrive pacing compared to CPAP in patients with obstructive sleep apnoea syndrome. Eur Heart J 2005;26(23):2568–75.

[31] Pepin JL, Defaye P, Garrigue S, et al. Overdrive atrial pacing does not improve obstructive sleep apnoea syndrome. Eur Respir J 2005;25(2):343–7.

[32] Simantirakis EN, Schiza SE, Chrysostomakis SI, et al. Atrial overdrive pacing for the obstructive sleep apnea-hypopnea syndrome. N Engl J Med 2005;353(24):2568–77.

[33] Sharafkhaneh A, Sharafkhaneh H, Bredikis A, et al. Effect of atrial overdrive pacing on obstructive sleep apnea in patients with systolic heart failure. Sleep Med 2007;8(1):31–6.

[34] Hanly PJ, Zuberi-Khokhar NS. Increased mortality in patients with Cheyne-Stokes respiration in patients with congestive heart failure. Am J Respir Crit Care Med 1996;153(1):272–6.

[35] Lanfranchi PA, Braghiroli A, Bosimini E, et al. Prognostic value of nocturnal Cheyne-Stokes respiration in chronic heart failure. Circulation 1999;99(11):1435–40.

[36] Cohn JN, Levine TB, Olivari MT, et al. Plasma norepinephrine as a guide to prognosis in patients with chronic congestive heart failure. N Engl J Med 1984;311(13):819–23.

[37] Solin P, Kaye DM, Little PJ, et al. Impact of sympathetic nervous system activity in heart failure. Chest 2003;123(4):1119–26.

[38] Lanfranchi PA, Somers VK, Braghiroli A, et al. Central sleep apnea in left ventricular dysfunction: prevalence and implications for arrhythmic risk. Circulation 2003;107(5):727–32.

[39] Ponikowski P, Chua TP, Piepoli M, et al. Chemoreceptor dependence of rhythms in advanced heart failure. Am J Physiol 1997;272:H438–47.

[40] Kushida CA, Littner MR, Morgenthaler T, et al. Practice parameters for the indications for polysomnography and related procedures: an update for 2005. Sleep 2005;28(4):499–519.

[41] Wexler L, Javaheri S. Sleep apnea is linked to heart failure, but does treatment improve outcome? Cleve Clin J Med 2005;72(10):929–36.

[42] Franklin KA, Eriksson P, Sahlin C, et al. Reversal of central sleep apnea with oxygen. Chest 1997;111:163–9.

[43] Andreas S, Weidel K, Hagenah G, et al. Treatment of Cheyne-Stokes respiration with nasal oxygen and carbon dioxide. Eur Respir J 1998;12:414–9.

[44] Staniforth AD, Kinnear WJ, Starling R, et al. Effect of oxygen on sleep quality, cognitive function, and sympathetic activity in patients with chronic heart failure and Cheyne-Stokes respiration. Eur Heart J 1998;19:922–8.

[45] Mak S, Azevedo ER, Liu PP, et al. Effect of hyperoxia on left ventricular function and filling pressures in patients with and without congestive heart failure. Chest 2001;120(2):467–73.

[46] Javaheri S. Pembrey's dream: the time has come for a long-term trial of nocturnal supplemental nasal oxygen to treat central sleep apnea in congestive heart failure. Chest 2003;123(2):322–5.

[47] Nakayama H, Smith CA, Rodman JR, et al. Effect of ventilatory drive on carbon dioxide sensitivity below eupnea during sleep. Am J Respir Crit Care Med 2002;165(9):1251–60.

[48] Javaheri S. Acetazolamide improves central sleep apnea in heart failure: a double-blind, prospective study. Am J Respir Crit Care Med 2006;173(2):234–7.

[49] Javaheri S, Parker TJ, Wexler L, et al. Effect of theophylline in sleep-disordered breathing in heart failure. N Engl J Med 1996;335(8):562–7.

[50] Marino PL. The ICU book. 2nd edition. Baltimore (MD): Williams & Wilkins; 1998.

[51] Naughton MT, Rahman MA, Hara K. Effect of continuous positive airway pressure on intrathoracic and left ventricular transmural pressures in patients with congestive heart failure. Circulation 1995;91:1725–31.

[52] Naughton MT, Benard DC, Liu PP, et al. Effects of nasal CPAP on sympathetic activity in patients with heart failure and central sleep apnea. Am J Respir Crit Care Med 1995;152(2):473–9.

[53] Tkacova R, Rankin F, Fitzgerald FS, et al. Effects of continuous positive airway on obstructive sleep apnea and left ventricular afterload in patients with heart failure. Circulation 1998;98: 2269–75.

[54] Kaneko Y, Floras JS, Usui K, et al. Cardiovascular effects of continuous positive airway pressure in patients with heart failure and obstructive sleep apnea. N Engl J Med 2003;348(13):1233–41.

[55] Sin DD, Logan AG, Fitzgerald AS, et al. Effects of continuous positive airway pressure on cardiovascular outcomes in heart failure patients with and without Cheyne-Stokes respiration. Circulation 2000;102(1):61–6.

[56] Bradley TD, Logan AG, Kimoff RJ, et al. Continuous positive airway pressure for central sleep apnea and heart failure. N Engl J Med 2005; 353(19):2025–33.

[57] Kohnlein T, Welte T, Tan LB, et al. Assisted ventilation for heart failure patients with Cheyne-Stokes respiration. Eur Respir J 2002;20:934–41.

[58] Teschler H, Dohring J, Wang Y, et al. Adaptive pressure support servo-ventilation: a novel treatment for Cheyne-Stokes respiration in heart failure. Am J Respir Crit Care Med 2001;164: 614–9.

[59] Philippe C, Stoica-Herman M, Drouot X, et al. Compliance with and effectiveness of adaptive servo ventilation versus continuous positive airway pressure in the treatment of Cheyne-Stokes respiration in heart failure over a six month period. Heart 2006;92:337–42.

[60] Pepperell JC, Maskell NA, Jones DR, et al. A randomized controlled trial of adaptive ventilation for Cheyne-Stokes breathing in heart failure. Am J Respir Crit Care Med 2003;168:1109–14.

SLEEP
MEDICINE
CLINICS

Sleep Med Clin 2 (2007) 119–123

ELSEVIER
SAUNDERS

Index

Note: Page numbers of article titles are in **boldface** type.

sleep.theclinics.com

Moving?

Make sure your subscription moves with you!

To notify us of your new address, find your **Clinics Account Number** (located on your mailing label above your name), and contact customer service at:

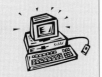

E-mail: elspcs@elsevier.com

800-654-2452 (subscribers in the U.S. & Canada)
407-345-4000 (subscribers outside of the U.S. & Canada)

Fax number: 407-363-9661

Elsevier Periodicals Customer Service
6277 Sea Harbor Drive
Orlando, FL 32887-4800

*To ensure uninterrupted delivery of your subscription, please notify us at least 4 weeks in advance of move.